# COMBATING THE CRISIS: EVALUATING EFFORTS TO PREVENT VETERAN SUICIDE

## HEARING

BEFORE THE

## COMMITTEE ON VETERANS' AFFAIRS
## U.S. HOUSE OF REPRESENTATIVES

ONE HUNDRED FOURTEENTH CONGRESS

SECOND SESSION

THURSDAY, MAY 12, 2016

## Serial No. 114–68

Printed for the use of the Committee on Veterans' Affairs

Available via the World Wide Web: http://www.fdsys.gov

U.S. GOVERNMENT PUBLISHING OFFICE

25–157                    WASHINGTON : 2017

For sale by the Superintendent of Documents, U.S. Government Publishing Office
Internet: bookstore.gpo.gov   Phone: toll free (866) 512–1800; DC area (202) 512–1800
Fax: (202) 512–2104   Mail: Stop IDCC, Washington, DC 20402–0001

# COMMITTEE ON VETERANS' AFFAIRS

JEFF MILLER, Florida, *Chairman*

DOUG LAMBORN, Colorado
GUS M. BILIRAKIS, Florida, *Vice-Chairman*
DAVID P. ROE, Tennessee
DAN BENISHEK, Michigan
TIM HUELSKAMP, Kansas
MIKE COFFMAN, Colorado
BRAD R. WENSTRUP, Ohio
JACKIE WALORSKI, Indiana
RALPH ABRAHAM, Louisiana
LEE ZELDIN, New York
RYAN COSTELLO, Pennsylvania
AMATA COLEMAN RADEWAGEN, American
  Samoa
MIKE BOST, Illinois

CORRINE BROWN, Florida, *Ranking Member*
MARK TAKANO, California
JULIA BROWNLEY, California
DINA TITUS, Nevada
RAUL RUIZ, California
ANN M. KUSTER, New Hampshire
BETO O'ROURKE, Texas
KATHLEEN RICE, New York
TIMOTHY J. WALZ, Minnesota
JERRY McNERNEY, California

JON TOWERS, *Staff Director*
DON PHILLIPS, *Democratic Staff Director*

Pursuant to clause 2(e)(4) of Rule XI of the Rules of the House, public hearing records of the Committee on Veterans' Affairs are also published in electronic form. **The printed hearing record remains the official version.** Because electronic submissions are used to prepare both printed and electronic versions of the hearing record, the process of converting between various electronic formats may introduce unintentional errors or omissions. Such occurrences are inherent in the current publication process and should diminish as the process is further refined.

# CONTENTS

## Thursday, May 12, 2016

# COMBATING THE CRISIS: EVALUATING EFFORTS TO PREVENT VETERAN SUICIDE

---

**Thursday, May 12, 2016**

COMMITTEE ON VETERANS' AFFAIRS,
U. S. HOUSE OF REPRESENTATIVES,
*Washington, D.C.*

The Committee met, pursuant to notice, at 10:00 a.m., in Room 334, Cannon House Office Building, Hon. Jeff Miller [Chairman of the Committee] presiding.

Present: Representatives Miller, Brown, Lamborn, Takano, Bilirakis, Brownley, Roe, Titus, Benishek, Ruiz, Huelskamp, Kuster, Coffman, O'Rourke, Wenstrup, Rice, Walorski, Walz, Abraham, McNerney, Radewagen, Zeldin, Costello, Bost.

## OPENING STATEMENT OF JEFF MILLER, CHAIRMAN

The CHAIRMAN. The Committee will come to order. Good morning, everybody. Thank you for being with the Committee for today's Oversight Hearing entitled, "Combating the Crisis: Evaluating Efforts to Prevent Veteran Suicide."

As the hearing title suggests, we are here this morning to discuss the ongoing veteran suicide crisis that, according to the latest data available from the Department of Veterans Affairs finds 22 veterans a day dying at their own hands.

I am disappointed that the VA was not able to release updated veteran suicide statistics at this time for this hearing. I understand that the Center for Disease Control finally provided national data to VA in the middle of March. Considering the critical interest in updated veteran suicide data, I can't emphasize enough the need for VA to pursue their analysis with a sense of urgency.

It is my fervent hope that the new data will show a reduction in the rate of veteran suicides as a result of the investments we have made in VA mental health care and suicide prevention. Regardless, I am hopeful that VA's witnesses today will be able to provide some more recent insights into the numbers of veteran suicides, and to shed some light on whether the efforts dedicated to this crisis are indeed making any impact.

I recognize the challenges that VA, and indeed the American health care system as a whole faces in preventing suicides. The rates of suicides have risen significantly over the past 15 years for almost every single demographic except for veterans, and I think that is due in large part to the hard work that VA health care providers do every day to extend helping hands to those most in need, but that is not to imply that the current rate is in any way acceptable.

I continue to be concerned that, again, according to the latest data from VA that is admittedly dated, the number of veterans dying by suicide has not fallen despite significant increases in budget, in staff and programming for VA mental health care, and a number of targeted veteran suicide prevention initiatives. It is not enough for veteran suicide rates to remain stable, our work will not be over until veteran suicide rates are eliminated.

There are many reasons a person may choose to take their own life, and there are many opportunities along the way for someone to step in and to intervene. VA should certainly be proud that veteran suicide rates have not risen along with rates in the general population, but there is clearly a deadly disconnect between the many services and supports that VA offers and the veterans that most need our help.

Care, particularly for someone that is contemplating suicide, is not one-size-fits-all. And while suicide undoubtedly is a mental health issue, it is also much more than that. Eliminating veteran suicide all together will take a comprehensive approach to ensure that those most at risk have not only the care they need, but also a job, a purpose, and a system of support in place to help carry them through their struggles.

Therefore, VA must adopt a suicide prevention strategy that recognizes the need for wraparound services, that treats patients as individuals, and embraces complementary and alternative approaches to care where appropriate.

Furthermore, VA needs to better integrate a veteran and family perspective that incorporates the lessons learned from those who have been on the front lines of the fight against suicide, and can offer a personal perspective and a message of hope to those that are still struggling today.

Last year, the Clay Hunt Suicide Prevention For American Veterans, or SAV Act, was signed into law. This law was named after a brave, 28-year-old Marine, Clay Hunt, who returned from battle against our enemies in Iraq and Afghanistan, but who in 2011 lost his personal battle to the demons he brought home with him from those conflicts.

The law included a number of provisions that I believe will help connect veterans in crisis with the care that they need both in VA, and in their communities that will provide valuable information about what programs are working for veterans in crisis, and assist VA in recruiting high-quality mental health professionals to treat veteran patients. Fully implementing the Clay Hunt SAV Act should be VA's highest priority.

I look forward to discussing the Department's progress to date and hearing about how the implementation of that important legislation is helping VA's efforts to prevent suicide among our Nation's veterans. In Clay's memory and in the memory of the countless other veterans who have lost their lives to suicide, we have to do better.

With that, I yield to the Ranking Member, Ms. Brown, for an opening statement that she may have.

## OPENING STATEMENT OF CORRINE BROWN, RANKING MEMBER

Ms. BROWN. Thank you, Mr. Chairman, for calling this hearing today.

Strong oversight of the Department suicide prevention program remains a priority of this Committee. We are all aware of the often-cited statistics of 22 veterans a day committing suicide. We also note that VA reports in 2014 that there is a decreased rate of suicide among users of the Veterans Health Care System with mental health conditions. The question becomes how can we ensure ready access to safe, quality mental health services to veterans in need of care.

I hope that the VA witnesses here today will be able to update us on those numbers, as much of the country was not included in previous estimates.

My subject that concerns me relates to the new MyVA 12 breakthrough priorities. I understand that addressing the suicide problem is not one of those. Increased access to health care, improving comprehensive and pension exams, continue to reduce homelessness, and transform the supply chains are all on the list, but specifically reducing suicide is not included. Given that suicide nationally is considered by some to be a public health problem, I believe VA should include suicide prevention as number one of MyVA priorities.

I look forward to VA testimony on this and where suicide prevention fits into the 12 priorities. I still believe that suicide prevention should be one priority of their own, top priority.

This hearing will also examine and implement the Clay Hunt Suicide Prevention for American Veterans Act, passed in the early days of the 114th Congress. This law focused the Nation on this terrible epidemic affecting veterans. This law requires that the Secretary of Veterans Affairs and the Secretary of Defense arrange for an outside evaluation of their mental health care and suicide prevention. It also requires any servicemember being discharged to have their case reviewed for any evidence of post-traumatic stress disorder or trauma, brain injury, or military sexual trauma.

We have been at war for over 14 years, there are many veterans out there who do not engage the VA care system for purposes of mental health treatment, veterans from all era. Today the discussion should include how VA is going to reach out to these veterans.

And I definitely want to say that one of the major problems, and I thank the VA for having the conference on suicide prevention that I was able to attend, but one of the points that was pointed out that many of the veterans, even though we have 22 a day, only three of them are involved in the system, and many of them are Vietnam veterans who when they returned home, wasn't received properly. So we need to figure out how we are going to reach out to these veterans and include them in the system.

And with that, Mr. Chairman, I yield back the balance of my time.

[THE PREPARED STATEMENT OF CORRINE BROWN APPEARS IN THE APPENDIX]

The CHAIRMAN. Thank you very much, Ms. Brown.

With us this morning is Dr. Jackie Maffucci, the Research Director for the Iraq and Afghanistan Veterans of America; Joy Ilem, the National Legislative Director for the Disabled American Veterans; Thomas Berger, the Executive Director of the Veterans Health Council for the Vietnam Veterans of America; and Kim Ruocco, the Chief External Relations Officer for Suicide Prevention and Postvention for the Tragedy Assistance Program for Survivors.

And we are also joined by Dr. Maureen McCarthy, VA's Assistant Deputy Under Secretary for Health for Patient Care Services, who is accompanied by Dr. Harold Kudler, VA's Chief Consultant for Mental Health Services, and Dr. Caitlin Thompson, VA's National Director for Suicide Prevention.

Thank you all for being here today to testify before our Committee.

Dr. Maffucci, you are recognized for five minutes.

## STATEMENT OF DR. JACKIE MAFFUCCI

Dr. MAFFUCCI. Thank you. Chairman Miller, Ranking Member Brown and Committee Members, on behalf of IAVA, thank you for the opportunity to share our views on this critical issue.

In 2014, IAVA launched the Campaign to Combat Suicide, a result of our members continually identifying mental health and suicide as the number-one issue facing post-9/11 vets. This campaign centers around the principle that timely access to high-quality mental health care is critical in the fight to combat suicide.

The signing of the Clay Hunt SAV Act into law was an important first step. We thank Richard and Susan Sulky for courageously inspiring us all to do the right thing, Congress for passing this legislation, and the VA for their commitment to fully implement the law.

We knew it would take time, and we are pleased that we have been included in the process. We are committed to working with the VA, Congress and our VSO partners to progress both the SAV Act and new initiatives that are certain to follow.

Personally, I have been working on this issue for about eight years and never in that time have I seen a movement around this issue so strong or a collective will so unified than in this last year. The conversations are moving to action, and it is our responsibility to make sure that this continues.

So today I would like to focus on four specific areas critical to progress: access to care, interdisciplinary approach to care, supporting those most at risk, and the importance of research.

In IAVA's annual member survey, over 80 percent of members with a mental health injury reported seeking care. This is an increase from our last survey. They continue to emphasize the role of the family and friends with over 75 percent who reported having a loved one suggest they seek help and, as a result, getting that help.

For those in care, three of four of our members are using the VA. This year, we saw over 75 percent of those using VA mental health services report little to no scheduling challenges, which is up ten percent from last year and comparable with those using a non-VA clinician. The same number were also satisfied with that care. But with more help seekers comes more demand, and it is critical to ensure that the VA is properly resourced to provide this high-quality care.

Efforts are under way with the Administration to bolster the VA workforce, recruiting medical students and improving curricula, but that is not enough. Beyond the challenge of a clinician shortage is the difficult task of hiring and retaining talent in the VA. The Federal hiring process is confusing and lengthy, at times deterring or rejecting qualified candidates; it must be made easier.

The VA needs to fully understand why staff are leaving. They need to know how best to attract and retain talent, and to use updated staffing models and real-time data to establish where the need is. Climate surveys are showing that in large part, VA is losing staff because of noncompetitive salaries and low morale. We all play a role in workforce morale at the VA.

We often forget to praise the dedicated staff who support VA's mission, some of whom are IAVA members. Our members have shared stories of the great work and dedication of these staff, relaying how these individuals saved their lives or cared for them in some of their hardest moments. We all must do our part to help celebrate what makes the VA good, while also focusing on how to make it better.

Finally, we need to ensure that high-quality care exists outside VA. Just under 40 percent of the veteran population actually seeks care at VA, which means the current community clinical workforce needs to be equipped to support veterans and their families and our recent-ran report suggests this is not the case. It is not even common practice to ask a military history, this has got to change. But beyond asking about military histories, community care doctors need to know how best to provide treatment once they have the answer, and the VA and its academic partners are best equipped to lead this effort.

But it is not just about mental health care. In February, IAVA and VVA called upon the Secretary to elevate the VA's Suicide Prevention Office, and we are pleased that that call was answered. While mental health is a major aspect of suicide prevention, it is not the only aspect. There are social factors that impact this as well.

For the VA Suicide Prevention Office to truly take a public health approach to decreasing suicide, it must have impact wherever veterans and their dependents go. Within VA, this has to include VBA. So we ask Congress to ensure that the office, the Suicide Prevention Office is fully resourced through a line item on the budget, so that it can be certain to carry out its critical mission.

We have also been focused on veterans with bad paper. This is a community that has been identified at high risk for suicide and homelessness. We can do something about this. IAVA urges passage of the Fairness for Veterans Act as part of the solution, but we also know that we together need to come up with a comprehensive solution with Congress, DoD and VA.

And yet with all of this, we simply don't know enough yet, and this is where the research piece comes in. We know that suicide impacts seniors disproportionately, but we don't know why. We know that women vets have a high rate of suicide, but don't understand how best to intervene. This is why IAVA supports the House-passed Female Veterans Suicide Prevention Act, and calls on the Senate to take immediate action on the bill. We know that the post-9/11 generation are showing an increased risk, but are just starting to understand the risk factors to impact interventions.

More research and evaluation is critical to developing these interventions. We simply cannot solve what we don't understand.

The VA has a wealth of research and a wealth of data, and they need to call upon academics to partner with them. And so we are asking the VA to open up their data and invite academics to help be their army to look at this data and help us find the solutions.

All veterans deserve the very best our Nation can offer. We look forward to working with Congress and the Administration to address these very real challenges with informed solutions.

Thank you.

[THE PREPARED STATEMENT OF DR. JACKIE MAFFUCCI APPEARS IN THE APPENDIX]

The CHAIRMAN. Thank you very much, Doctor.

Ms. Ilem, you are recognized for five minutes.

### STATEMENT OF JOY J. ILEM

Ms. ILEM. Thank you, Mr. Chairman. We appreciate the opportunity to testify as well on this important issue.

Over the past decade, VA has enhanced and promoted a comprehensive set of mental health services, including integration of mental health into primary care, and a goal of improving access, minimizing barriers and reducing stigma.

Research shows early intervention and timely access to mental health care are key to improving quality of life, promoting recovery, obviating long-term health consequences, and minimizing the disabling effects of mental illness and the risk of suicide.

In recent years, VA's mental health programs and suicide prevention efforts have been both praised and criticized. Outside sources have described the scope, depth and breadth of VA's multivariant mental health approaches as superior to care in the private sector. Additionally, data shows that VA users have a lower suicide rate than veterans not using the VA Health Care System, as you have noted. However, there have been documented issues with access in the past, over-prescribing of medications and serious failures for some veterans, along with a call to action to do more to prevent suicide in this population.

In our opinion, VA has two major challenges. One, to ensure it meets the diverse needs of an increasing number of veterans, enrolled veterans, who need specialized mental health services and, two, how to effectively outreach to veterans who are not using VA, but are in crisis or in need of help.

Younger veterans indicate they prefer a variety of nontraditional therapies over medication, such as Web-based life coaching, yoga, meditation, and acupuncture. While VA is steadily increasing the availability of these non-medical approaches, there is still variability of access to complementary and alternative services across the system.

This past weekend DAV, along with a group of community-based organizations, sponsored a Spartan Weekend for ill and injured veterans, centered on the promise that they would not take their own lives without reaching out to someone for help. The event reached 1.8 million Facebook and other social media users, and resulted in a number of veterans reaching out for help for the first time.

We believe these types of community events will be essential for connecting non-VA users to the mental health services they need.

Another challenge VA faces is how to ensure veterans with war-related mental health issues get quality care in the community through the Choice program. While DAV prefers VA to be the provider of specialized mental health services whenever possible, immediate access to care is the most critical factor for a veteran in a mental health or emotional crisis.

This group can particularly benefit from VA's peer-to-peer program, its expertise in treating PTSD, substance use disorder, and TBI, as well as the wraparound services and other post-deployment transition challenges they often face.

If a veteran with mental health issues needs to access care in the community, we urge VA to routinely follow-up with the veteran to ensure the patient is receiving quality and effective care from a provider with expertise in treating veterans with war-related or sexual trauma.

Another area we recommend VA put focus on is crisis management. When a veteran is experiencing a mental health crisis and asking for help, there must be ready access for mental health services. We are pleased in that regard that VA has been working to improve training and services through its crisis line and pilot new programs for peer specialists, who have been found to be very effective in helping to coach veterans into care and keeping them in care.

Another area we urge focus on is women veterans. According to VA, the suicide rate is six times higher for women veterans compared to civilian women. Increased suicide rates are also reported among women who have experienced military sexual trauma. However, it is encouraging to learn that women veterans who use VA health services were 75-percent less likely to die by suicide than women veterans who did not use VA. This data suggests that VA's mental health programs for women, including suicide prevention efforts, are showing promise and positive results, and that a concerted focus on this subgroup of veterans should be continued.

We do, however, suggest that there be improved access for women veterans to specialized in-patient and residential mental health programs to ensure recovery and effective reintegration. VA must ensure all of its mental health programs meet the unique needs of women, including safety and privacy concerns.

In closing, we urge VA to continue its training and partnerships with the community providers, improving its mental health programs and research on suicide prevention, and to find innovative ways to engage all veterans who need specialized mental health services. We ask Congress to do their part as well, providing VA with the resources to address expansion of mental health programs, their recruitment challenges, staffing issues, and ongoing research.

It is our hope that as a community, we can work together to ensure that any veteran who needs help can get it.

Mr. Chairman, that concludes my statement. Thank you.

[THE PREPARED STATEMENT OF JOY ILEM APPEARS IN THE APPENDIX]

The CHAIRMAN. Thank you.

Dr. Berger, welcome, and you are recognized for five minutes.

## STATEMENT OF THOMAS BERGER

Mr. BERGER. Thank you, Chairman Miller and Ranking Member Brown, and distinguished Members of the House Veterans' Affairs Committee.

Vietnam Veterans of America thanks you for the opportunity to present our testimony regarding the Department of Veterans Affairs efforts to reduce suicide among the veteran population.

The timing of this HVAC hearing is particularly important, as some of you may have read the recent National Center for Health Statistics report that found that suicides in the United States has surged to the highest levels in nearly 30 years, with increases in every age group except for older adults in the age group, both men and women, over the age of 75. The overall suicide rate has risen by 24 percent from 1999 to 2014, according to that report, and the increases were so widespread that they lifted the Nation's suicide rate to 13 per 100,000 people, the highest since 1986.

There is absolutely no doubt that this country is in the midst of a public health crisis with suicide and nowhere is that any more true than in the veterans community, as we learned back in February, 2013 with the VA's report on veterans who die by suicide. In particular, that report painted a shocking portrait of what is happening amongst our older vets, my cohort and those who served before me, because almost three quarters of the veterans who commit suicide, based on that report, are age 50 or older, according to that report.

And even though suicide has become a major focus for the military over the last decade, most research by the Pentagon and the Veterans Affairs Department is focused on men, who account for more than 90 percent of the Nation's 22 million former troops, little has been done or focused on female veteran suicide until recently.

According to an L.A. Times article in July, 2015—and by the way, I have to apologize, my written testimony says July, 2016, I can't read into the future, and I need to get my auto correct fixed on my machine— anyway, the suicide rates are highest among young female veterans for women ages 18 to 29. Veterans kill themselves at nearly 12 times the rate of non-veterans.

And according to that same Times article, amongst that cohort that was looked at, the suicide rate of female veterans closely approximate that of male counterparts, in effect, women vets at 28.7 per 100,000 versus 32.1 per 100,000 male vets.

But we also can't forget, as the Chairman has alluded, that it is from that 2013 report that the figure of 22 veteran suicides per day is calculated. This number is suspect because of the data only representing numbers reported from 21 states from 1999 through 2011 and did not include states with massive veteran communities like California and Texas, which didn't report their suicides to the VA at the time.

Therefore, VA calls for an updated veteran suicide report that includes data from all 50 states and U.S. territories, and also we strongly suggest that VA mental health services develop a nation-wide strategy to particularly address the problem of suicides amongst our older veterans. Now, obviously I am speaking on behalf of our Vietnam Veteran-era group.

At the same time, we understand it is very challenging to determine an exact number of suicides, but we have got to overcome the barriers, identify and overcome the barriers that prevent our servicemembers from seeking the help that they need and that they deserve.

VVA is heartened in particular by the efforts the VA has made since February, 2016, including those efforts that were mentioned by Dr. Maffucci earlier. While these initiatives are laudable, VVA also believes strongly they cannot be fully successful without a significant increase in the recruitment, hiring and retention of VA mental health staff, as well as timely access to VA mental health clinical facilities and programs, especially for our rural veterans. And this Committee is in a position that can ensure that our veterans and their families are given access to the resources and programs necessary to stem the tide of veteran suicide.

Once again, on behalf of VVA's national officers, board and general membership, thank you for your leadership and holding this important meeting, and I will be glad to answer any questions.

[THE PREPARED STATEMENT OF THOMAS BERGER APPEARS IN THE APPENDIX]

The CHAIRMAN. Thank you.

Ms. Ruocco, you are recognized.

## STATEMENT OF KIM RUOCCO

Ms. RUOCCO. Chairman Miller, Ranking Member Brown and other distinguished Members of the Veterans' Affairs Committee, the Tragedy Assistance Program for Survivors, TAPS, thanks you for the opportunity to share stories from surviving family members of servicemembers and veterans who have died by suicide.

These families are honored to have a voice in this process and they gain healing from the thought that this testimony in remembrance of their loved one may in fact save a life.

My name is Kim Ruocco and I am Chief External Relations Officer for Suicide Prevention and Postvention for the Tragedy Assistance Program for Survivors. Following my husband's death, I joined together with Bonnie Carroll and TAPS to build a comprehensive peer-based support program for all those who are grieving a death of an active-duty servicemember or recent veteran who had died by suicide.

TAPS' ultimate goal is to help these families of the fallen to rebuild their lives on a solid foundation of hope, healing, love, and a new sense of belonging after a death by suicide. TAPS presently has over 7,000 suicide survivors from the military and 700 survivors of military murder-suicide.

For the purpose of today's testimony, I have gathered information from family members who have recently lost a veteran to suicide. Survivors of military suicide hold a wealth of information on the multiple factors that lead up to this kind of death. They are on the front lines of a servicemember or veteran's battle with PTS, DBI, mental illness, moral injury, and the multiple stressors associated with military life. They are witness to the challenges of stigma associated with mental health and the barriers to care for those who are suffering. Survivors of veteran suicide loss can provide us with a picture of potential impact of challenges within the VA system. Today's testimony is a summary of information gathered from these families.

The first common theme was barriers to care. It is important to note that in each case, that I have highlighted the veteran was not in ongoing, consistent, evidence-based treatment at the VA. In most cases, the veteran struggled to get the care they needed in a timely fashion. In some cases the veteran himself or herself was the first barrier to good care because of their cultural beliefs, their stigma regarding mental health. This reluctance to share their true story, fear that they would not be believed or insistent that they need to push through and suck it up, in combination with institutional barriers, can become a perfect storm for those veterans that are suffering.

Families of these veterans struggled to help their loved one and often became frustrated and overwhelmed with navigating the system. Many of them express frustration with the lack of their involvement in the assessment and treatment of their loved one. They claim that part of the veteran culture is to not complain or admit to emotional and physical pain, and to downplay how serious their issues actually are. Families feel strongly, if they were present for intakes and evaluations, they would have had a more accurate diagnosis and treatment plan. Most families state that it was difficult to get the veteran to go and agree to get help, and then when they did go, it was usually during a crisis period and there was long waits or inability to see someone at that time, or a misunderstanding of their struggles or a missed diagnosis.

The second theme that was throughout all of our families' conversations was the quest for peer support. In each case, the family tells TAPS that the veteran only wanted to talk to someone else who had been there. The veteran had a lot of shame and guilt about the symptoms they were feeling, and thought that these symptoms were a weakness in them and not an illness. This false belief became a barrier to getting timely, appropriate treatment.

Peer support can be used to build trust and eventually leads to an understanding that their symptoms are real and valid, and that there is treatment that works. Peers serve as a beacon of hope that those who are struggling could offer a roadmap to navigating the system.

So here are our recommendations based on our findings. We have to increase the number of mental health providers that are trained in evidence-based best practices for treatments of these injuries and illness. At each contact, a veteran should be able to get appropriate mental health care in a timely manner, and this is especially true in crisis points like ERs, outpatient clinics and primary care.

Two, the families would love to develop advocacy and information groups that can offer support and guidance for those who are supporting a veteran, so they can get answers.

Number three, develop an avenue for family members to call for professional advice and get guidance on symptoms, treatment, and how to get their loved one into care.

Four, make peer support specialists a line item. Peer support is an invaluable tool and reciprocal relationship that adds value to all involved. Peer support specialists can be used to reach out to these veterans where they are and build a bridge towards treatment and help them stay in treatment.

And finally, five, increase incentives for and streamline process for peers to become mental health professionals. In the case of veterans, personal experience adds a level of trust and credibility that greatly increases the probability of a veteran seeking treatment and staying in treatment.

Thank you so much for listening to us today. We have many families that came to me and would like their stories heard, and we have those available to you, if you would like to hear them in the future.

Thank you very much.

[THE PREPARED STATEMENT OF KIM RUOCCO APPEARS IN THE APPENDIX]

The CHAIRMAN. Thank you very much for your testimony.

Dr. McCarthy, you are recognized for five minutes.

### STATEMENT OF DR. MAUREEN MCCARTHY

Dr. MCCARTHY. Good morning, Chairman Miller, Ranking Member Brown and Members of the Committee. Thank you for the opportunity to discuss the effectiveness of the Department of Veterans Affairs mental health programs and our efforts in preventing veteran suicide.

I am accompanied by Dr. Harold Kudler, Chief Consultant for Mental Health, and Dr. Caitlin Thompson, National Director for Suicide Prevention.

VA has developed the largest integrated suicide prevention program in the country. We have over 800 dedicated and passionate employees, including suicide prevention coordinators, Veterans Crisis Line staff, epidemiologists, and researchers who spend each day preventing suicide and caring for veterans.

Our overarching strategy enhances veterans' access to high-quality mental health care and implements upstream programs designed to help veterans before they consider suicide. Veterans who reach out for help must receive that help when and where they need it in a way that makes sense for each of them.

We do have a good story to tell today, one in which we wish to share hope and progress, and in which we want all veterans to know that VA is here to help, but the rest of the story is, we still have work to do. We are pleased to share our progress and the opinions of others outside of VA about the quality of our efforts.

On February 2nd, we hosted a summit on "Preventing Veteran Suicide: A Call to Action," to bring together veterans, families, other Federal agencies, community partners, veteran service organizations, subject matter experts, Members of this Committee, and other key partners to enhance our work on suicide prevention.

Powerful for so many attendees were the stories shared by veterans and their families. These stories truly resonated with us.

Just as we don't prevent sudden cardiac death only when it is happening, we know that suicide prevention does not necessarily begin with our crisis line or other interventions when suicide is imminent. Our efforts are about hope, finding reasons for living, leading a high quality life, and developing strong, meaningful relationships. Engaging veterans in VA care, and in particular in our whole system of care, is a key part of prevention. Addressing their job concerns, substance abuse, homelessness, financial concerns, general medical health, and of course mental health are all important steps in preventing suicide.

The Call to Action generated multiple recommendations and initiatives to strengthen VA's approach to suicide prevention. For example, a pilot project is underway to evaluate risk-intervention strategies based on data that predict who would be at risk for suicide before these individuals reach a crisis.

Also, VA continues to actively monitor suicide-related behaviors through our Suicide Prevention Applications Network. We are working to develop a dashboard that will allow us to identify possible clusters of suicide-related behaviors, and to trigger meaningful responses or interventions.

VA remains committed to ensuring the safety of veterans, especially when they are in crisis. We do have universal access for 24/7 emergency care through our emergency departments and by VA's Veterans Crisis Line. The program continues to save lives and link veterans with effective ongoing mental health services on a daily basis.

Preventing suicide also requires access to mental health care, as our partners on the panel have noted. Between 2005 and 2015, the number of veterans who receive VA mental health care grew by 80 percent, a rate of increase more than three times that of the overall growth of VA users. This reflects VA's concerted efforts to engage veterans new to our system and stimulate better access to mental health services. We remain committed to eliminating the stigma associated with receiving mental health care. In 2007, we rolled out integrated mental health services in primary care clinics, which allow veterans to receive warm handoffs from their primary care team to a mental health provider present in the primary care clinic on that same day.

VA has also moved to patient-centered community care, a centralized contracting mechanism, and has implemented the Choice program. We are addressing access through our efforts such as extended hours to help increase capacity and the hiring over 900 peer specialists, while expanding their role into primary care settings.

We partner with more than 150 mental health organizations around suicide prevention. We recognize that we cannot do this alone, and we continue to develop and prioritize these partnerships.

We are aware that some veterans are at an even greater risk of suicide. We have individual and group-specific interventions tailored to help these high-risk veterans. Of course, any risk for any veteran is one we must continue to address.

VA has taken steps to implement each of the requirements of the Clay Hunt Suicide Prevention for American Veterans Act, including our Call to Action. VA has contracted with an independent third party to conduct evaluation of mental health and suicide prevention programs, we are collecting self-report outcome data from veterans newly receiving mental health care, we are working towards release of a Web site that provides easily accessible information about all the mental health services for veterans. Currently, the VA facility locator tool is accessible on several sites, including VA's home page. It includes contact and resource information for a variety of mental health programs.

Mr. Chairman, the crisis of suicide among veterans mobilizes us to continuing and expanding upon the work we have done. We remain focused on providing the highest quality of care for our veterans while trying to understand more about precursors of suicide among veterans. We appreciate the support of Congress, those at this table and all partners in our mission, and we will be happy to respond to any questions you may have.

Thank you.

[THE PREPARED STATEMENT OF DR. MAUREEN MCCARTHY APPEARS IN THE APPENDIX]

The CHAIRMAN. Thank you very much, Doctor. You talked about having contracted a review of your suicide-prevention programs and other outreach efforts. When do you expect to receive the final product from that review?

Dr. MCCARTHY. So the contract is with the Enterprise Resource Performance, Incorporated, they have started their work. I think we are due to give you a report by August about what is happening with the report, but in two years their review will be complete.

The CHAIRMAN. So it is a two-year program, but we get an interim report hopefully in August?

Dr. MCCARTHY. Yes, sir.

The CHAIRMAN. Okay. When we are on our summer work period.

Dr. MCCARTHY. We will happily do it whenever is convenient.

The CHAIRMAN. As soon as possible. Thank you.

Can you also talk to us about the vacancies that exist, what your current vacancy rate is right now in health care? And then, I think it is important for the Committee to know and to understand what is the total time that it takes from recruitment all the way through to bringing a mental health provider on board right now at the VA.

Dr. MCCARTHY. I have to say, I am not the person that knows the exact number of days it takes from recruitment. I can tell you the process and that it does likely take several months.

When asked about the actual vacancy rate of psychiatrists, I believe Dr. Shulkin testified before this Committee we were at about 236. We are working—

The CHAIRMAN. Out of how many? 236 out of?

Dr. MCCARTHY. Harold, do you know the number of psychiatrists we have? I have it in my notes somewhere.

Mr. KUDLER. I believe it is about 800.

Dr. MCCARTHY. About 800. And as we continued to hire and expand, some moved around and then we had vacancies. There is turnover in mental health. The psychologists, there is a lower rate of vacancy, I don't have the number.

The CHAIRMAN. Go ahead and talk about the process of recruitment going all the way through to bringing somebody on board.

Dr. MCCARTHY. So typically there is advertisement, people apply, often through USA Jobs. The applicants are reviewed, interviews are conducted. There is a credentialing process that is sensitive to how quickly information is imported into the credentialing process, it is usually a minimum of two weeks, but it can take up to a month or two depending on the delays. We have worked to streamline helping providers get the information they need in there relatively quickly. After that, an offer is made and a start date is given.

I do not have the average time and I would be happy to get back with you on that.

The CHAIRMAN. Okay. And we talked a little bit about the Clay Hunt—

Dr. MCCARTHY. Yes, sir.

The CHAIRMAN [continued]. —Suicide Prevention Act and according to the figures that I have, because of the enrollment period being extended, there have been almost a thousand veterans that have been enrolled into the VA Health Care System. What have you learned from those roughly 995 individuals in regards to your outreach to them, and what can be done to provide more information about current programs?

Dr. MCCARTHY. Thank you, sir. The question really is not just what we learn from them, but also other veterans as well that have chosen not to come and see us. What we learned also as part of the Call to Action, part of the Clay Hunt implementation, was people want us to make it easy for veterans who are leaving the military to enroll in VA health care.

So we have worked with DoD, and we have begun a process currently ongoing with our Health Eligibility Office to try and decrease any barriers to help, that every person leaving the military have a health plan when they leave. We have done that especially already for people that have been engaged in mental health care, but now this is for all of them to have a health care plan when they leave.

And so what we are looking at is not automatic enrollment, but essentially close to that. So that if they haven't chosen or indicated another health care system, we would like to decrease any bureaucracy or any barriers for them receiving health care and get them enrolled in VA very quickly.

The CHAIRMAN. What are the biggest barriers that you have heard that they feel like they have to overcome to get into the system?

Dr. MCCARTHY. On some level, there is a sense that some veterans do not understand that they are entitled to care. And for our vets who are post-9/11 who are leaving, there is that five-year eligibility window, there really should be no barrier. We have treated women veterans who said literally in a clinic, I didn't know I was eligible for services.

And so we have to change our messaging to be more welcoming to all of our veterans. As much as we try, we have people at outreach events, our suicide prevention coordinators do five outreach events a month, we go to the welcome home and the yellow ribbon ceremonies and so forth, but something is not happening where people are not understanding that they are eligible or else they are choosing not to come.

The CHAIRMAN. Thank you.

Ms. Brown?

Ms. BROWN. I will go with the Committee and then I will go last. So the person, who is the first person?

The CHAIRMAN. Mr. Takano?

Ms. BROWN. Yes.

Mr. TAKANO. Thank you, Mr. Chairman.

Mr. Chairman, I want to thank all the witnesses for your testimony, I also want to make a pitch to you, Mr. Chairman. Mr. Coffman held a wonderful reception for a group of people from Colorado that did a wonderful video, in which you are partly featured, and I hope that we can do something to encourage the Committee as a Committee to take the time to view that. It goes very deep into the topic of PTS. And I hope that you might, with encouragement, with help from Mr. Coffman and Mr. Perlmutter, do that.

The CHAIRMAN. Why don't we do this, I will spring for the pizza and we will have a showing of that here in the Committee room in the very near future. I haven't seen it, but I understand it is very, very good.

Mr. TAKANO. It is very good, very powerful. It is long, but I think it will give Committee Members other ideas that we need to follow and follow through on.

The CHAIRMAN. Well, the director, Stefan Tubbs, is a very impassioned advocate.

Mr. TAKANO. Well, certainly I intend to show it at events in my district, and it is a very bipartisan video.

Anyway, I have some questions for, I believe it is the VA, about TAPS. I understand that TAPS is a big supporter of peer-based counseling, and you recommended in testimony that peer support specialists should be a line item in the budget. What do you recommend that VA do better with regard to their peer support program?

Ms. RUOCCO. Well, I know there is about 900 out there now, but there needs to be more. We need more money to get that program built bigger, and to have them everywhere, because what our families told us, is that they had a lot of trouble getting their veteran to the VA. They had a lot of misconceptions about what would happen there, they don't understand treatment, they are afraid of treatment, they are afraid of being over-drugged. And so they would not go to the VA until they were in crisis, and then it is very difficult to get immediate mental health care when you are in crisis, where we would rather have them in the system before the crisis getting treatment.

So these peer specialists have done everything from going and finding a homeless veteran, to bringing them to the VA and getting them into the system, to getting them housing, to sticking with them and describing what treatment is. To saying I went there, I had the same symptoms, I went there and I am better.

So they can really be a bridge for all of this, because I think one of the biggest challenges is not getting our veterans who are suffering into good, evidence-based treatment for the things that they are suffering with these wars.

And all of my cases are ones who fell through the cracks, they all died by suicide. And every one of them that I talked to had tried to go to the VA, had tried little places, but they didn't go until they were in crisis and then it was very difficult to get the treatment they want when they are already in crisis, and so many things had already interfered with their lives.

Mr. TAKANO. Dr. Berger?

Dr. BERGER. I think it is misleading to say that, generalizing and say 900 peer-support persons have been hired, it makes it seem like they are all in mental health when that is not true. Okay? So I think we need some answers about how many peer-support people do we actually have in mental health.

Mr. TAKANO. Is there a response to that question?

Dr. MCCARTHY. So the number that we quoted are primarily mental health or they are part of the primary mental health integration program. So they are linked to being the ones that reach out and encourage the veteran to receive care.

Mr. TAKANO. Do we need to fund this more, do we need to fund more? How much more do we need to fund it?

Dr. MCCARTHY. Is that for me, sir?

Mr. TAKANO. Yes.

Ms. RUOCCO. In my understanding, there is two pieces, right? There is the peer support specialists that are the training, but then there is also an avenue for peers to become mental health providers, right? That is two separate things. So having peers, veterans who have been there, get the training to be mental health counselors in the system is a win-win for both, because we are taking those veterans who had this experience and were able to use it to do good and to save other veterans.

So it is two different tracks. We are talking about peer support specialists to go out in the community and get them into the VA, and we are talking about a streamline of getting peers, veterans trained in mental health to be counselors, two separate pieces.

Mr. TAKANO. Okay. My question is, is there adequate funding and, if not, how much more do we need?

Dr. MCCARTHY. I don't have that, but we would be happy to get back with you on that amount.

Mr. TAKANO. Please. Thank you.

Dr. MCCARTHY. Thank you. Could I just clarify the number that I gave as the number of vacancies? I am sorry, Chairman Miller.

We currently have 5,500 on-board psychologists and 3,200 on-board psychiatrists in VA. And so when I talked about 236 vacancies, it is 236 out of 3,203.

The CHAIRMAN. Okay.

Mr. Lamborn, you are recognized.

Mr. LAMBORN. Thank you, Mr. Chairman, and thank you for having this important hearing today.

Dr. McCarthy, the bill that we passed, the Clay Hunt Suicide Prevention Act for American Veterans, requires the VA to collaborate with nonprofit mental health organizations to do three things to improve the efficiency of suicide prevention efforts, to assist other nonprofit organizations to do a better job and to collaborate with these nonprofit organizations. What is the VA doing and how are these collaborative efforts coming along?

Dr. MCCARTHY. So I did mention before our Call to Action summit that happened in February, that is one piece of it. We really brought a lot of people together, not for us to tell them, but for them to tell us what we really need to be doing, what we need to keep doing, what we need to do better, what we should do differently.

More than that, we sponsor community mental health summits around the country and this is the fourth year of doing it. Each medical center sponsors a summit in which information is shared bidirectionally. Our homeless outreach folks have done that and mental health has been doing that. We have learned and we have shared, and it has been extremely productive for the collaboration.

One other thing we have been doing is actually working with partners in the community who provide care. We realize that, especially as part of Choice, there are veterans that are out there receiving mental health care and we want them to have a warm welcome reception in the community, just like we want for them to have that at VA.

We have developed in partnership with DoD a military competence training for providers. It provides up to eight hours of continuing medical education free for community providers or internally, for people to be able to understand the language, and about taking a military history. We have also lobbied to have a CPT code added for taking a military history, which is part of a reimbursement mechanism in the private sector, so that people will be encouraged and financially rewarded for doing that.

Mr. LAMBORN. Okay, thank you.

And, Dr. Berger, I would like to ask you a question about research. And I think we all agree, there needs to be more research. You said that about 70 percent of veteran suicides are people, among males, is people of the age 50 and older and, according to your chart, 85 percent of male veteran suicides are age 40 or older.

Mr. BERGER. Well, sir—

Mr. LAMBORN. So my question is, my question is, let's say Vietnam-era veterans who served 40 to 50 years ago, let's say between '65 and '75, 1965 and 1975, tell us about the connection between that service and a suicide at the age of 70 or something like that. And I understand probably every suicide is for unique and personal reasons, but what does research tell us about the connection there?

Mr. BERGER. Well, certainly there are risk factors that all veterans share. There is no denying it. But at the same time, as we age, there may be additionally risk factors added to the pool.

For example, in the case of our older vets, it may involve insurance, health insurance kinds of things, if they are not enrolled in the VA in particular. There may be family issues that surface at that time. The structure in our lives changes, but at the same time, I am not aware of any focus, gerontological research on these different aged cohorts and which risk factors may be important at particular points in time.

Mr. LAMBORN. Thank you. And I appreciate the work of every one of you on the panel. Our hearts go out to those who have committed suicide at whatever age. And so thank you for your preventative work.

Mr. Chairman, I yield back.

The CHAIRMAN. Thank you, Mr. Lamborn.

Ms. Brownley, you are recognized.

Ms. BROWNLEY. Thank you, Mr. Chairman.

And I wanted to thank Dr. Maffucci for bringing up the Female Veteran Suicide Prevention Act, and I am encouraging all of you to help in supporting this bill. We have a companion bill in the Senate, and I certainly would like to see this particular piece of legislation see it through. Because I think the focus, although Dr. Berger talked about, I believe you talked about an increase in being able to treat women veterans, I think it is really critically important that the VA is the expert, the absolute expert in this issue around suicide and particularly looking at best practices for both our male and female veterans, because I do think a female experience on the battlefield can be very different from a man's experience. So thank you for that.

I also, you know, wanted to talk a little bit about the outreach. And I know that we have a transitional program to have a warm handoff when our veterans leave the service from the DoD to the VA, and I think that that is positive. I am curious to know how well that is going and what it looks like, but I think we have to actually dig back further.

In other words, you know, it seems to me we should have medical professionals on the battlefield there. I think in terms of outreach with family members, I think we need to, for a veteran who is sent to the battlefield, who is potentially going to experience trauma, the family members should be trained and prepared, so on their reentry back, the family members need to know.

And when we talk about older veterans, which for the first time today I am aware that the suicide rate amongst older veterans are going up, you know, we have got to figure out some kind of outreach in those cases as well.

But I do think, you know, we train our men and women to go to the battlefield and be prepared to save their physicality and their physical health, but we also need to prepare them to survive their mental health as well. And so I think we have to go further back starting really at the beginning, so that people are knowledgeable and aware, and even the veteran can be aware of their own behaviors and help themselves.

So I guess, you know, the question that I would like to get some answers from is, you know, really how this handoff situation from the DoD to the VA is really working. How do these handoffs take place, what are they looking like, and are we collecting some data on that to figure out if this kind of warm handoff is actually working?

I open it up to anyone.

Dr. BERGER. I will jump right in here, at least from the perspective of what I know about it.

You know, VVA has stayed away from using the term "seamless transition," because there is no such thing. I would only point out we have many, many cases where the transfer, quite frankly, there is no other way to say it, is screwed up, and it ends in the result, focusing on today's topic, in a veteran's suicide.

For example, I am sure you have all heard, there is at least two or three cases in the last year or so of vets who were prescribed certain kinds of medication, and DoD for their mental health challenges, they get to the outside, those records weren't forwarded to the VA, or there was some kind of barrier or what have you. The

VA gives a diagnosis, puts them on perhaps another complete set of mental health medications, and they can't cope and they take their own lives.

Ms. BROWNLEY. Dr. McCarthy, do you have any responses in terms of that response and how you believe the program is working? And if what Dr. Berger is saying is true, how do we rectify that?

Dr. MCCARTHY. So I will be happy to respond to the medication parts, and I will turn it over to Dr. Thompson about the program, if that is okay. Thanks, Tom, for bringing that up.

We have had an opportunity to look very closely in our cross-agency partnerships about this particular transition time and medications. And we have made it now so that all psychiatric and pain meds that would be prescribed in DoD could be prescribed in VA, and it is our expectation that the medications would continue seamlessly. However, the expectation is that the provider would do a safety review. So if, for instance, there are multiple drugs of the same class and too many, that at that point, they could be adjusted. But the expectation clearly is that this go well.

We started, we have done two sets of chart reviews, actually looking at specifically transitioning veterans. Of a thousand veterans that we checked, I believe the number was 20 that had a medication change that was not what we expected it to be. That is 20 too many. And so we have provided feedback to those providers who made that change, we have also increased our education program specifically about meds.

But I would like Caitlin to talk about the transition program.

Ms. BROWNLEY. Well, my time has run out, but maybe we can follow-up.

I yield back, Mr. Chairman.

The CHAIRMAN. Thank you.

Dr. Roe?

Mr. ROE. I will yield my time to answer the question.

Dr. THOMPSON. Thank you, sir.

So we also have what is called the In Transition Program, which is a coaching model so that servicemembers who have difficulties with mental health are given a coach while they are still in service, who then help them and make sure that they have that transition point across to the VA. But we really take all of this extremely seriously, especially because we know, and for older veterans, but also for others, that those veterans who are going through transition in any way are at very high vulnerability for suicide risk.

Mr. ROE. Thank you.

I want to start by first of all thanking the VA. I think you all have, I think you do have the largest comprehensive mental health program in the United States and it is not perfect, but it is certainly better than it was seven years ago when I first got here, seven and a half years ago. There is no question the focus that the Congress have given and the VA has given has improved things.

One of the things that is hard to do in suicide, first of all, as a practicing physician, was to identify those people who are at risk, because it is a silent demon you carry around and you don't share with anyone. And I think one of the things that we have learned today is, is that when patients, veterans do get into care at the VA, their suicide rate goes down. I think we have figured that out.

Number two, I think we have also learned that the hiring process at the VA is ridiculously long and should be shortened for not just mental health, but other providers of health care. I think that has got to be shortened and I don't know what takes so long. I have hired multiple physicians in my career and it doesn't take that long. It is not that hard to do to do your background checks and so forth to find out what you need.

I think the other thing that has been brought up, and what is confusing about this, is when you look at the data and I think the cohorts of people are different. For instance, us guys, Vietnam-era guys, that is a different cohort than the younger veterans that are leaving. And when you look at the suicide data from 2001 to '07, non-deployed veterans had suicide rates higher than deployed veterans, which is confusing for us. I mean, why does that happen? So I think more research is important.

And I think one of the things that we have to do, the family and friends, there is no question, I looked at data years ago when I was in practice that showed that somebody who went to a psychiatrist had a higher rate of suicide than somebody who talked to their best buddy. So having a good friend to talk to someone and having someone, as you pointed out very clearly, I think you need to expand this program where you can touch a buddy that was in the service. Those of us who have served have a different look at things, a view of the world and so forth, and when you have somebody that has put their overalls on just like you have, it makes a big difference. And I think that is a program that works and it should be expanded.

The other thing I want to encourage you to do at VA and outside the VA is good, good data, because without that you can't make the right decisions, you just cannot. And you can't group us all into one big group, you have got to look at different cohorts. We are female, younger veterans and older veterans like I am.

So I will stop there and let anyone make a comment.

Dr. McCarthy. So maybe I could mention the data analysis that is going on right now, because we are excited about this. This is very different from what we did in the past where we had to get data from the states and some states gave us data and some did not. We have worked with CDC and with DoD and have requested data on everybody that had been in the military or the VA between 1979 and 2015. And so we sent multiple discs with data that could be matched with the CDC data for suicide. And it is coming back to us, it is very raw. It involves a lot of individual checking and so forth. We so wanted to have the data to share with you at the hearing, we don't. We were told that it would be analyzed by the middle of the summer, and we promise we will get it to you as soon as we can.

But we are really excited, because this is not state-specific and it crosses ages, sexes and all those other kind of risk factors that we really want to be able to identify. And we want to make that data available to our academic partners in a transparent way, so others can help us understand the data.

Mr. ROE. A few things that were said, and Dr. Berger pointed it out, that this 22, you just saying 22, well, that is probably not correct. Because if you look, it was just 21 states, it probably isn't correct, and yet that is quoted all the time. That is why we need accurate data.

And in the U.S., we are 50th in the world in suicide, and I am proud of the fact that we are really pointing it out, because it all comes down to one person. Look at all this data, it doesn't matter when you are the one person, the one patient out there, the one veteran or civilian that is contemplating taking their life. It is preventable. It is just like opioid addiction and deaths, those are preventable deaths if we pay attention.

I yield back, Mr. Chairman.

The CHAIRMAN. Thank you very much.

Ms. Kuster, you are recognized.

Ms. KUSTER. Thank you very much, Mr. Chair. And thank you, Dr. Roe, for setting up my comments on the opioids, because as I sit and listen—and by the way, this is one of the best panels I have heard since we have been here, but as I sit and listen, there are so many corollaries. I am a co-chair of the bipartisan Congressional task force to combat the heroin epidemic, and we now have over 80 bipartisan members and we are passing 15 bills this week. And I want to commend my colleagues on both sides of the aisle and Jackie Walorski for her work on veterans. We passed yesterday the Promise Act. But there are so many corollaries and many of the same people, four out of five heroin users have a co-occurring mental health disorder, often undiagnosed and untreated.

But I wanted to speak to you particularly, Ms. Ruocco. First of all, my condolences for your loss, but thank you for your courage.

Ms. RUOCCO. Thank you.

Ms. KUSTER. And a big part of this is about stigma, it is about mental health generally, and the stigma around mental health. So one piece that I want to convey to you is that we want to help, help you to be a leader on addressing stigma and particularly for veterans.

In New Hampshire, I am very proud of a new program that we have that is called, "Ask the Question," and we are using this across the state. This is way beyond the veteran community, this is our entire health care community, mental health community, every person that comes in contact with anyone who comes before them to ask the question, did you ever serve?

My father was a World War II pilot. He was shot down, he was a POW for six months, no one ever asked him this question. He never talked about it until he was well into his 70s and it was only when my boys growing up started asking him all the questions. What was the plane like? What happened to you? What do you mean, what happened after you hit the ground? You know, tell this story.

So I am curious about this peer support, because this is what one of my communities has just started for heroin use and it turns out that incredible psychological bond of someone who has been before you, and if you could talk more about how can we help you to grow that program.

And then, just generally for any of the witnesses, how can any of us here help with the stigma and the support?

And then just lastly, I really want to commend a candidate and I don't mean this to be partisan, to be honest, I don't even know his party, but this is in yesterday's Politico, "One Candidate's Risky Bet Talking About his PTSD," he is running in Delaware and he is a veteran. And it is a risky bet, but the courage for you as a family member to come forward and for others to come forward I think is critical.

Ms. RUOCCO. Thank you so much. And I am from Massachusetts, so I am aware of that campaign and it is a great campaign.

And we actually have all been speaking together, like Caitlin and I work a lot together on messaging with the Department of Defense, and one thing we have really talked about is, there is a need for all of us as a whole to change the messaging around the VA and around suicide.

Ms. KUSTER. Good.

Ms. RUOCCO. You know, that number 22 that has been going around, we had a suicide in the veteran population about five months ago who left a suicide note and in the suicide note said, I am going to be one of the 22 today, why should I even try? So having the negative messages out there that it is an epidemic, that there is 22 dying a day is increasing hopelessness in our veteran population and the feeling of helplessness and the feeling that treatment doesn't work. It is the biggest barrier to them getting real, good treatment with the demons that they are bringing with us from, you know, unresolved early childhood trauma and additional combat-related issues.

So I think we need a campaign where we are all speaking with one voice about the people that are getting treatment, that treatment works, that more people are getting treatment and surviving than are dying by suicide. So that we can get those veterans out there really thinking, you know what, there are others that have gone through this, they have survived it, and they are doing well. Because we have amazing veterans in our communities that are doing unbelievable work, and we have peer-based programs all over the country like Red, White and Blue and Team Rubicon that are pulling these veterans together, are providing hope and are real beacons of who these veterans really are. They are loyal and they are smart and they are dedicated.

So we have got to start a campaign that looks at that and talks about that, and stop focusing on the fact of how many have died. We have raised the awareness, we know it is a problem, let's get in the forums like this and fix the problem, but at the same time, get a message going out there that treatment works and it doesn't have to be that way.

So I think that is really—

Ms. KUSTER. Well, my time is up. I am sorry, we will have to come back on another round. But I would just say, I saw the other night on television this Invictus that is going on this week—

Ms. RUOCCO. Yes.

Ms. KUSTER [continued]. —with the sports. It is so powerful, the hidden wounds of war. And this is part of what we are going through in the addiction community is anonymity has been such a big part of this, which is important for treatment, but for those on the other side to come out and start to tell their story—

Ms. RUOCCO. Yes.

Ms. KUSTER [continued]. —is so powerful. So thank you so much for being with us.

Ms. RUOCCO. So powerful. Thank you.

The CHAIRMAN. Thank you very much.

Dr. Benishek, you are recognized.

Mr. BENISHEK. Thank you, Mr. Chairman. I too would like to thank you all for being here this morning.

I just want to follow-up on something with Dr. McCarthy that has been bugging me since I have been around here. I don't know, I mean, is it emblematic of what is going on, is it a sign of the sincerity of the VA? But I have an issue with when you call the VA hospital and there is an automated message that says dial 1 for the pharmacy, dial 2 for the outpatient clinic, dial 3 for the OR, but if you have a mental health crisis, please hang up and dial a ten-digit number. Okay? Well, this is a pet peeve of mine. All right?

And I have been working on this, and now only in my district they fixed that. All right? Because I have been on it all the time. But as of this morning, in Michigan, the Iron Mountain VA and the Saginaw VA have fixed it, but there are still three Medical Centers in Michigan that you have to hang up and dial an 800 number.

Now, I brought this up in Committee a long time ago, and I am asking why this is not fixed. And they said, well, it will all be fixed in six months. Well, that was more than six months ago. And I would like to know why we just can't fix this right now? Why does this change take so long?

You agree it should be fixed, right?

Dr. McCARTHY. Oh, sir, absolutely.

Mr. BENISHEK. Is there anybody—

Dr. McCARTHY. I have good news. Do you want some good news? There are 12 VAs where you can press 1 and get directly connected from the Medical Center—

Mr. BENISHEK. Twelve.

Dr. McCARTHY. Twelve, to the crisis line.

Mr. BENISHEK. That is what I am telling you, that is not very many.

Dr. McCARTHY. Including Hawaii and a few other places, which is pretty great in terms of the technology. It is not all of them, and it should be all of them. And that is clearly in the works and—

Mr. BENISHEK. Yeah, but you see, this is why I bring this up. Okay? Because to me this is something that should be just fixed automatically, without taking a year to do it. All right?

So here we are talking about mental health crisis. All right? And you can't do this. Do you understand what I am saying? We have got all kinds of huge problems to solve in dealing with mental health patients and you can't fix this? It is outrageous. I mean, I am amazed by this.

I mean, it hurts me, because these are blocking and tackling, this is solving the individual problems that veterans have when calling. This is a crucial thing. I mean, I have had individuals talk to me about this very problem, you know, and they try to kill themselves in the parking lot of the VA because they couldn't get help.

So what I am trying to tell you in my comment here is that this is a blocking-tackling minor thing, these are the kind of things you have got to fix every day and not take a year to do it.

So you are telling me that there are only 12 places in the country that this is actually occurring out of the hundreds of VA facilities around?

Dr. McCarthy. It is my understanding it was 12 the last time I checked. I know that it is rolling out really quickly.

Mr. Benishek. Is there somebody within the VA that is resisting this change that you are aware of?

Dr. McCarthy. Oh, no. We have a rather old phone system, and we have a number of challenges with it, but I am not trying to—

Mr. Benishek. Well, don't give me that. You have got the dial 1 for the pharmacy, it connects to the pharmacy just fine.

Dr. McCarthy. Okay.

Mr. Benishek. You know what I mean?

Dr. McCarthy. Right.

Mr. Benishek. So don't blame it on the phone system.

Here is the other thing I want to know. When you dial this crisis line, I mean, a lot of people end up dialing the crisis line because that is the only place they can get a person, right? So what is the process for triaging people that call the crisis line who may not actually be in mental health crisis, but they are just trying desperately to talk to somebody at the VA?

Dr. McCarthy. So let me let Dr. Thompson take that call, because she has worked there.

Dr. Thompson. Thank you, sir. These are such important points and I do want to—by the end of the summer, all of the VAs will have rolled out the press 7, so that those press 7 numbers get to the Veterans Crisis Line. The reason that they have to pilot it is because they have to know how many people will be available at the crisis line as they roll this out, otherwise there won't be enough people to answer those calls.

Mr. Benishek. So right now, you are saying the 800 number, there is nobody there?

Dr. Thompson. I am sorry, sir?

Dr. McCarthy. No, sir, no.

Mr. Benishek. Your answer makes me suggest that you are not rolling it out because you don't have people behind the scenes to do it.

Dr. Thompson. No, we have to—that is to pilot things, in order to understand what the rollout is going to be, but I assure you that by the end of this summer all the VAs will be rolled out. But we absolutely understand—

Mr. Benishek. That was what you said last year.

Dr. Thompson [continued]. —and hear your concerns. This has taken longer than we had thought and—

Dr. McCarthy. We personally tested it and—

Mr. Benishek. What about the question I just asked about the—

Dr. Thompson. Yes, sir. So when people—and I worked in the crisis line for five years—when people call the crisis line, there is a set of questions to ensure that the person isn't at immediate risk and needing somebody right away, which happens 30 to 40 times a day where somebody needs that immediate help because they are in the process of dying by suicide, they can't commit to being safe. So but—

Mr. BENISHEK. How many questions is it?

Dr. THOMPSON. I mean, it varies as far as there are certainly a few questions that are important—

Mr. BENISHEK. How long does it take?

Dr. THOMPSON [continued]. —for a suicide risk assessment.

Mr. BENISHEK. How long does it take?

Dr. THOMPSON. To do a suicide risk assessment?

Mr. BENISHEK. On the phone, yeah.

Dr. THOMPSON. The immediate question is, are you safe right now, really, and that is an immediate question. And then there needs to be developed a rapport with the person who is calling. So many of the people that call, this is the first time—

Mr. BENISHEK. All right, okay.

Dr. THOMPSON [continued]. —they have called before—

Mr. BENISHEK. I am out of time. Thank you.

The CHAIRMAN. I will be glad to give you some more, if you need it.

Dr. THOMPSON. And I am happy to keep answering the question, but—

The CHAIRMAN. Well, unfortunately, I don't know your answers are what he is looking for, you know. I mean, to talk about a silly pilot on something as serious as this is just ridiculous.

Mr. O'Rourke?

Mr. O'ROURKE. Thank you, Mr. Chairman.

And, Mr. Chairman, I would like to begin by thanking you for bringing much needed attention and focus and accountability to this issue. I can't think of a more important issue for us to be working on, and I think that is reflected in your leadership. And I would just ask that we continue to keep the pressure, and the focus and our commitment to provide the resources and the oversight necessary to make progress on this issue. And I think to a person we are all there with you and the Ranking Member to maintain this as a priority.

And I want to thank everyone who is part of the panel today from the VA and from the advocate community, for your help and focus, the information that you are bringing to this, so that we can make better decisions, so that we can hold ourselves and the VA accountable for making improvements.

And I want to echo the Ranking Member's suggestion that, through you, Dr. McCarthy, this goes to the Secretary, he has 12 wonderful priorities for transformation of the VA, not one of them is specific to reducing veteran suicide. And I authored a letter that the Ranking Member, Republicans and Democrats signed asking for just that. I would hate to have to do that legislatively. I think that is something that the Secretary can do and should do, and we will ask him through you to do just that.

Until it is a stated priority, we are not going to see the changes that we need to see; we are not going to prioritize prevention, we are not going to move from pilot programs to full implementation of necessary interventions. I just believe in that wholeheartedly, and it needs to happen. And if we need to get the veterans advocate community behind that to create the political pressure and will to do that, then so be it, but let's not have to do that.

One of the questions I have, is whether we will just use the 22 as our baseline statistic, 22 veterans a day taking their lives, if 17 of those veterans are not accessing VA care and if we believe that if they were to have access to VA care the outcomes would have been better, Dr. McCarthy, is the VA ready today in terms of capacity, number of providers, space, other considerations, to see those 17 veterans?

Dr. MCCARTHY. That is a very thoughtful question. You know, what we have tried to do with the 17 is find other ways to have us reach out to them, and so we have this suite of mobile applications, we have worked on helping providers treat them and so forth. Space is a challenge.

Mr. O'ROURKE. So let me ask this, because I was really looking for a yes or no, and it sounds like the answer is no. I won't put words in your mouth. If the answer is in fact yes, tell me, but the answer it sounds like is no.

What I want to know, and you may not be able to answer it today, so I will take it for the record, but I will ask it at the next hearing if I don't get it before then, I want to know what it will take to be able to see each one of those 17 veterans, in terms of resources, in terms of planning, in terms of new facilities, in terms of agreements with community providers to take some of the pressure off the VA for what I would call non-core priorities. Arthritis is incredibly important to provide care for, so is diabetes, so is the flu, but if there is a community provider who can see veterans for those issues so that we can focus our hiring and our resources and our care for, as Dr. Roe said, an eminently preventable condition, suicidal ideation and ultimately suicide, then we should do that. I mean, we can prevent the loss of life. I can't think of anything more important for the VA to do.

So my question to you and through you to the Secretary, and I think each of us wants to see the answer to this, what will it take to see each of those 17 veterans?

Now, it sounds like we are going to have an updated number this summer.

Dr. MCCARTHY. Yes.

Mr. O'ROURKE. And so the question follows, if that number is 25 and only four of those 25, we want to know what the other 21 are going to do. So would you mind providing an answer, a full, detailed, accurate, honest answer to every Member of this Committee?

Dr. MCCARTHY. I would be happy to do my best to get that answer to you, sir.

You know, I took it when you asked me the question, did we have the capacity internally, and we do not have that capacity internally. When you mentioned community providers, we do have a network of community providers, but we are not up to speed with a hundred percent of them in that position.

So, yes, we will take your question, and I promise you, we will give you the answer to the best of our ability.

Mr. O'ROURKE. Thank you.

I yield back.

The CHAIRMAN. Thank you.

Mr. Huelskamp?

Mr. HUELSKAMP. Thank you, Mr. Chairman. I appreciate the opportunity to follow my colleague Mr. O'Rourke, who has done tremendous work on this, bringing it to the attention of the Committee and recognizing the difficulties in his area, which are not just there, but thank you.

And I want to follow-up a little bit more on those questions you mentioned and the network of community providers. Can you describe how the Choice program has worked in terms of mental health care and meeting the needs of rural areas like mine and elsewhere across the country?

Dr. MCCARTHY. So let me start with the Choice program. I can talk about the community care that was provided and the number of appointments that have been provided by Choice. I am going to speak in somewhat round numbers, but in fiscal year 2013 we had over 16,000 appointments in the community, in fiscal year 2014, 24,000. Fiscal year 2015, we had 31,000 in the community and over 3.4 thousand through Choice.

The Choice program has grown, this year we have over 18,000 so far, and there are a number that haven't yet been attributed to the year that when people were doing the review. So the Choice program is growing, and we are grateful for that, and I know our veterans are.

Mr. HUELSKAMP. And the numbers on Choice, do you know which those are based on, waiting too long versus distance requirements?

Dr. MCCARTHY. That, sir, I do not know.

Mr. HUELSKAMP. Okay. And do you have a general figure on the waiting time for those, and how do you calculate that in this particular situation?

Dr. MCCARTHY. So our under secretary has asked us to rethink access and how we talk about wait times and to do that in a veteran-centric way. He said really the only important measure of wait time is the veteran's satisfaction with how quickly they have been seen. And so that is the direction we are moving toward in calculating how we are doing with access. We have an online kind of—or a kiosk means, I am sorry, in which we will assess veterans each day as they are in our system, and did they get the care they needed when they felt they needed it.

And a similar question, we have what we use is the SHEP survey, and other health services systems ask the same questions as part of the CAP survey, but that question is, was the care available to you when you needed it? And that really is how we need to think about access in a veteran-centric way.

We want to be transparent, sir, and we just feel like as we have gone through all the descriptions of create date, desired date, you know, all those other descriptors, we have managed to confuse a lot of people, and really the most important person we want to satisfy is the veteran. And so our measures will—

Mr. HUELSKAMP. Well, in this situation, it is certainly not like other items in health care. We are dealing with suicide, obviously a very serious matter. I am not saying the others are not.

So what is the number? I heard the long description and how difficult. If you call and push 7, and you are one of the lucky 12

VAs—you don't have to dial the crisis hotline, how long does it take for you to see a mental health care provider? And do you not have that number or tell us.

Dr. McCarthy. So first of all, if you press 7 or you call the crisis line, that gets you to the crisis line where an assessment is made; "Is this an urgent situation?", just as was asked before. If the veteran is in urgent need and the veteran calls or comes to the medical center, our expectation is that that veteran is seen that day. Okay, they come to our emergency room, they are seen that day. An urgent need is seen that day.

However, if they come to a place like a community-based outpatient clinic and it is, you know, after hours or something and the clinic is closed, we need to understand urgency there. Our expectation is that the medical center, the parent medical center has an emergency room where that person could be seen. Urgent, same day.

Mr. Huelskamp. But what if you are 200 miles away?

Dr. McCarthy. So then, if you are working through the crisis line, the expectation is that the crisis line assists you with getting the care you need, reaching out either to the medical center, or to the suicide prevention coordinators in the medical center to arrange for that care. Urgent, the expectation.

Mr. Huelskamp. But, again, a little more. And these are limited circumstances, but in rural areas, I don't think you have the network in my area that you certainly have elsewhere. What do they do? I am just curious and maybe it is individual circumstances, each one of these probably, obviously is, but what do they do? When they are 200 miles away, they call the hotline, you say it is an urgent situation, what do you do next?

Dr. McCarthy. So Caitlin, who has worked the hotline, will explain this.

Dr. Thompson. Yes, certainly. And this happens all the time. The crisis line has received calls from people who are in the middle of lakes. And so, you know, you get that emergency personnel immediately to that person. If the VA is 200 miles away, they are going to immediately go to the closest facility, and all of that is coordinated between the crisis line and the local officials.

Mr. Huelskamp. Local officials? I am sorry to get into this, but unless the Choice program is working well, which in some cases it is not, you are just going to call—who would you call?

Dr. Thompson. So I think we may be talking about a couple of different things, but in terms of imminent situation, someone says I am feeling suicidal, the Veterans Crisis Line will get them to whoever is available at that moment, the closest person, and then they can coordinate that care afterwards.

Mr. Huelskamp. And I appreciate it. I am sorry, Mr. Chairman. Rural areas, and this is not just with veterans, this—where is the network? And I would be curious in the State of Kansas and elsewhere, show me who you would call, because I doubt that you have a network up that you could pick up the phone and say I know who to call out in the middle of western Kansas. And again, we are 200, 300 miles away, and in every other care, they are expected to drive until we did the Choice program.

So we could have some follow-up and discussion in my particular area, what do they do? Because I am hearing from veterans, I am hearing from folks that are active duty as well, what do they do?

Dr. THOMPSON. Yes.

Mr. HUELSKAMP. And, you know, the phone is not working in these emergent situations and long term as well, what do you do after that?

Dr. THOMPSON. Exactly.

Mr. HUELSKAMP. What do you do, you know, two months later and you are in some type, and there is not much of a network there?

Dr. MCCARTHY. And that is the crux of suicide prevention, so I will look forward to talking and follow-up.

Mr. HUELSKAMP. Okay. Thank you, Mr. Chairman. I apologize.

The CHAIRMAN. Thank you.

Miss Rice, you are recognized.

Ms RICE. Thank you, Mr. Chairman.

I am going to direct this question to Ms. McCarthy. I have heard from many veterans who separated from the military with what is called an other-than-honorable discharge, we all know that, that was their designation, and these veterans are often the ones who are the most difficult to reach out to, because depending on the discharge, they are not able to access many VA services like health care, housing or employment help.

The VA's characterization of the discharge process is, we all know, very messy. It often takes years before a decision is made on whether or not a veteran can have a reclassification so that they are eligible for these benefits.

And I want to just take a moment to thank our colleague Mike Coffman for introducing the Veteran Urgent Access to Mental Health Care Act, to ensure that all veterans, regardless of their discharge designation, can access the care they desperately need before something tragic happens. I mean, it seems to me that that is about as big a red flag as you can have for someone who might have suicidal issues because of that designation.

So what I want to know is, what is the VA doing specifically to increase outreach to this most vulnerable population of veterans with other than honorable discharges? Have you researched if there is a connection between that designation of other than honorable discharge and suicide or attempted suicides?

And I think your ability to kind of improve the characterization of discharge process is limited, because I know it is, you know, either Air Force or the specific wing, but what, if anything, have you done to address this issue?

Dr. MCCARTHY. So thanks for the question.

Let me start by saying that it is indeed a problem, and we have identified it certainly in partnership with IAVA. We have been working on trying to come to a solution. That is partly why we wanted to make sure, first of all, the mobile apps are all available. There is this whole suite of things where people can get help. They don't need to be enrolled as veterans, and yet they have access to these kinds of tools, the use of meditation, coaching for PTSD and so forth, online-type tools which can help them with their symptoms, help them identify them and then help them with the treatments.

We have vet centers which are able to follow a different set of rules for eligibility. Any Vietnam veteran seen, I believe, before 2004 at the Vet Center, and then all combat veterans are eligible for services at the Vet Center. There are—80 percent of the employees they are veterans themselves. And they can actually provide counseling for people regardless of the kind of discharge. And they also provide some counseling to active duty military.

As part of the Choice Act, we were asked to open our doors, and for active duty services members with MST, and some of them are coming to the vet centers for that kind of care.

Ms. RICE. What about the connection between the designation and suicides or attempted suicides?

Dr. McCARTHY. I—

Ms. RICE. Do you have that number or no?

Dr. McCARTHY [continued]. I don't have that. I think IAVA has that number.

Ms. RICE. Okay.

Dr. MAFFUCCI. So there has been a study done that suggests that those with bad paper are two times more at risk for suicide. And so this is one piece why IAVA has been so focused on this issue. There was a recent report out by Swords for Plowshares and some others that partnered on that report that estimates 125,000 post 9/11 vets with bad paper. Now, not all of these are going to fall into that category of needing mental health, but certainly some of them will. And for some of these, these are individuals who might have been received that discharge status due to symptoms of an undiagnosed mental health illness or injury.

And so this is why we have certainly urging passage of the Fairness for Veterans Act, but we are also calling for—we all need to come together. DoD—this is a DoD, VA, Congress and the VSOs and MSOs. There needs to be a comprehensive plan. We have been—over the last few years, there have been pieces that have been getting to the solution, but we haven't gotten near to that solution.

The other challenge is that many of the community providers out there, many of the community programs base their eligibility off of the definition and the eligibility requirements at VA. So even those programs that could potentially be helping these individuals aren't available to them.

The vet centers are fantastic. Our members are constantly holding them up as a top resources, resources they go to, resources they recommend. And one of the things we would like to see done is an assessment of the vet centers, how they are being used. Are there enough of them? Are they under utilized? Are they over utilized? And how can we expand them if they are being—if there is that demand there, because they certainly are not just for those with bad paper, but for families as well. I mean, their criteria is much more broad than the VA and they can do a lot more.

Ms. RICE. Ms. Ruocco, if I can just make a comment. I applaud you. I would imagine how difficult it must be for you to get past what must have been enormous anger, and for you to be able to deal with that and be sitting here and be such an advocate. I was at an event last night with an organization called PenFed. And they support obviously our veterans, but also last night, one of the caregivers for a veteran was given an award. And it was the mother of a servicemember who was severely wounded in his service. And I think it is time that we, you know, maybe focus on help to caregivers as well—

Ms. RUOCCO. Absolutely.

Ms. RICE [continued]. —because it is an enormous population that we ask a lot of and you sacrifice an enormous amount, and I thank you very much. Thank you, Mr. Chairman.

MS. RUOCCO. Well, thank you for that.

The CHAIRMAN. Thank you very much. Mr. Coffman, you re recognized.

Mr. COFFMAN. Thank you, Mr. Chairman. Appreciate the comments of Congresswoman Rice on this important issue of veterans being discharged under other than honorable conditions and being denied access to mental health care from the VA. Combat veterans with multiple tours of duty, who, I think in a very unfair way, for particularly the United States Army to conduct a reduction in force through singling out combat veterans who might have some disciplinary issues, oftentimes, we believe related to post-traumatic stress disorder, and that are discharged without any access to VA mental health care, is a recipe for problems in and of itself. And so this legislation and I know many of the Members here, Mr. O'Rourke, Mr. Walz, Mr. Zeldin and others are co-sponsoring this legislation. But we absolutely need to get that done. And I want to thank IAVA for being really a catalyst on this very important issue.

Let me just pivot to—I have a real concern that we have had testimony before this Committee before concerning a drug-centric therapy and form of treatment, modality of treatment. And in fact, we had testimony of veteran suicide where I think a former servicemember was given a cocktail of drugs in response to treatment. And then moved, relocated, the prescriptions ran out, was unable to navigate the bureaucracy of VHA to get those prescriptions refilled. And given the powerful nature of some of those drugs, took his own life.

And then, I think we have had testimony as well—well, in fact, I was with Congressman Lamborn in his district in Colorado Springs where we had testimony from parents of a Marine who had served tours of duty, I think in Iraq and Afghanistan, had left the service, went to the VA for mental health care. They gave him a very powerful drug that part of the directions on the drug were it required constant monitoring. He was not monitored. He subsequently took his life.

And so I just think that this reliance on these very powerful drugs is a shortcut to treatment by the VA. And I think it is costing veteran lives, and I want you to respond to that.

Dr. MCCARTHY. So, you know, I am not prepared to talk about individual situations, but I would be happy to talk about our expectation. When we had learned about some of these problems with people moving, we have made it really clear the expectation is that the meds continue, and that any barriers to that be broken down so that the meds would continue. So we appreciate that having been brought to our attention. And it is certainly our hope and our expectation that that particular problem is not occurring at this time.

As far as treatments go, the evidence based treatments for PTSD in particular include cognitive behavioral therapy, prolonged exposure therapies, all therapies that do not involve medications. And it is really important that the right kinds of treatments are used. As a provider, a psychiatrist, who has treated veterans with PTSD, I know that often the despair and the frustration and the impatience that you see when you talk to a veteran leads you to think I have got to do something. And I think that leads to people at times making choices about meds that they might not otherwise make. Let me try this, let me try that. You know, there is no single pill that is a cure for PSTD.

Mr. COFFMAN. Well, it becomes a pill to get up in the morning and a pill to go to bed at night.

Dr. MCCARTHY. Right. And—

Mr. COFFMAN [continued]. And a pill for this and a pill for that.

Dr. MCCARTHY [continued]. And that's why—

Mr. COFFMAN [continued]. And I think it has a very adverse cumulative effect. Let me also just mention that I think it has been brought—I think that it has been raised by this panel about the vacancies in the VA in terms of mental health providers being hired by VHA.

We had a very good roundtable with the leadership of VHA in this room not that long ago. And one thing that was interesting that was raised, in that was how difficult it is for somebody who wants a job, and the VA to navigate how long it takes to get accepted by the VA, and how long it takes to get placed by the VA, and how significant the attrition rate is by those who start the process and those who simply can't afford to finish the process. And so it has been raised that it is a function of compensation. I contend that it is part of this bureaucracy that needs to be cleaned up. Mr. Chairman, I yield back.

The CHAIRMAN. Thank you. Mr. Walz, you're recognized.

Mr. WALZ. Thank you, Mr. Chairman. And thank you to all of you for being here. And to the VA thank you on the Clay Hunt bill is near and dear to many in this room, not just up here or there, but those sitting behind you. And I appreciate the VA's not just approaching to fulfill the letter of letter of the law, but the spirit of the law. And for that you should be thanked and I am grateful.

Also I think the things that have been spoken by my colleagues talking about veteran health care in a vacuum outside of health care in general is the wrong way to go about this. I think in that lies an opportunity. We know the VA can't fix this alone. We know the private sector can't fix it alone. And certainly the veteran and the families can't fix it alone. That gives us the opportunity to find new ways to partner, new ways to deliver care, new ways to use best practices to move those things forward.

And I will echo what Mr. O'Rourke, the Chairman and the Ranking Member all said, and if I can add my word to this. It is obvious you have elevated this to the highest level. I think VA in general has to. When we see a list of 12 priorities, my suggestion is this better be near the top. That is why my constituents are asking for.

And in that I ask the question, I think we are asking, we have been tracking this very closely, this legislation, and there is no doubt in my mind that the willingness to implement it is there and it is happening. My question though is, it seems like the coordination might be something. And Dr. McCarthy, I don't question it, I just wonder and I ask you is, do we need to elevate VA suicide prevention office to the Office of the Secretary, is that the first step we need to do on this, just so that coordination is tighter?

Dr. McCARTHY. So thank you for that question. We are in the process of reorganizing the suicide prevention office and raising it higher in the organization right now, and increasing the number of staff, as well as the resources. When we talked about elevating it, at one point we did talk about a separate line item in the budget would effectively elevate it as well. But in any case, what we very much know is that it needs to report higher in the organization.

DoD has elevated it to the level of the Secretary. I'm not sure that is what we are going to do. Dr. Caitlin Thompson is our suicide prevention coordinator and we are having her report through the Under Secretary for Health, Dr. Shulkin. And I think that's an important place, given that in that position she will have the opportunity to reach across the aisle to VBA and effectively partner with DoD as we—

Mr. WALZ. Well, I certainly don't want us to interfere with the organizational structure down to that level, but I certainly do want everyone to know that, Dr. Thompson, I would like you to open up your office door to the Secretary on this one if that is what it takes to do this. That is what we are trying to do. And I would segue a little bit here to this next one. I think all of you have hit on this. It is the people we are not reaching, I think that is—I mean you do a wonderful job when we get them in. I think that is what many of the Members here are focused on.

New York Times reported on Clay Hunt's unit himself that that unit and the Minnesota National Guard, we are seeing clusters. We have got to get better at predicting these clusters and when they are happening. And I know that is tough stuff that you are all working on.

But I would say, and I ask about this, and the Chairman and the Ranking Member, all of you looking at this from a coordinated broader perspective, but there have been several mentions of groups that are actually doing this—of trying to get that coordination there, Team Rubicon and Jake Wood who served as battle buddy with Clay, those folks.

I would humbly request that we do something where we bring them in, sitting right where you are, to talk about how they are doing this, because there are groups like Team Rubicon and Ride Recovery and I mention, I am not singling out, these are folks that I have looked at, worked with, looking for evidence-based results on this. And the question that Mr. Huelskamp brought up is really good about building that network.

There is a headstrong group up in New York you may be familiar with working with Cornell University, they partner with the San Diego VA. And they said the San Diego VA is fabulous about saying "We can't handle all these. You guys need to help them." They built a network of the top psychiatrists and mental health people in the country. They are getting almost immediate care. It is incredibly cost efficient and they are out there and doing it. So that was our vision of the Clay Hunt. That was the vision of where these groups are at.

And I know Dr. Robrad (?) and the Centerstone people that operate in the Tennessee/Indiana areas. So I ask all of you, these are out there, they are doing it. Certainly what works for veterans is what works. We have to be evidence-based. We have to be cost conscious on how we will be delivering these. But the purpose of the Clay Hunt bill was get that peer to peer, get that out in the community. Do you feel it is happening? How much do you work with these groups? You know, you mention the names. We hear Team Rubicon. I just ask all of you quickly. I would like them to be here, because I think that model is a working one.

Dr. MCCARTHY. We fully agree and we do reach out. We are partnering with our folks at the table here often, and in addition with partners in the community. So yes.

Ms. RUOCCO. I would say that there are some really amazing things happening all over the country.

Mr. WALZ. Amazing.

Ms. RUOCCO. Like in Massachusetts the home-based program, which is taking in, educating, giving free treatment. And then there is like Vets for Warriors, who is peer based 24/7 call-ins. Those people are really, you know, bridging those gaps. So we have got to look at those, I think you are right, bring them in, what is working and really give them some funding to really expand.

Mr. WALZ. It goes back into that VA is the medical home—

Ms. RUOCCO. Yes.

Mr. WALZ [continued]. —of the coordinating center with Dr. Thompson. But using those groups almost rapidly and seamlessly.

Ms. RUOCCO. And support.

Dr. BERGER. Both Dr. Maffucci and I, in February, called for a strengthening of that coordination. And in fact, okay, Dr. Carolyn Clancy was named co-chair of the National Alliance for Suicide Prevention. Okay. And as a Member of the executive committee, there could be some stronger efforts by our VA partners in pushing that message out because they have got all those connections with some of the groups, most of the groups that you mentioned.

Mr. WALZ. They are building networks. I know my time is over. I just think there is a golden opportunity here. And it is not a critique on this. I think this is moving in a direction that many of us wanted to see. The seamless use, the building the networks, the reinforcing that. You are going to—we can streamline the hiring, we can do all that, that is not going to make all the difference though. Those folks are out there. So I thank you. Thanks, Chairman.

The CHAIRMAN. Mr. Zeldin, you're recognized.

Mr. ZELDIN. Well, thank you, Mr. Chairman. Dr. McCarthy, so I served four years on active duty. I have been in the Reserves since 2007. I have lost more people I have known in the service due to PSTD, than I have in combat. And it has impacted my home county pretty hard. I represent Suffolk County. We not only have the highest veterans population of any county in the state, we are second highest of any county in the country.

And there was some conversation earlier pretty much in your opening statements you were getting at peer support. And I just want to get an idea of what kind of a model you may be considering, if not doing already, as far as peer support groups.

Dr. McCarthy. So I would like to turn to Dr. Kudler to describe this.

Dr. Kudler. Thank you. VA has been hiring and training peer support specialists. It doesn't even—the 990 or so we have, doesn't include about 100 Global War on terror and outreach workers at vet centers, at the 300 vet centers around the country. And we train them to run groups, we train them to be in waiting rooms, to look for people who are agitated and anxious, and that includes primary care, as well as mental health. In some places, in emergency departments for instance, at the Phoenix VA, now has a peer support person in the ED to kind of hang out and wait for people who maybe—might want to walk out before their wait time ends.

And we are training them to do therapy. We are training them to help support clinical work like compliance with medication, to call people up and help. And by the way, we also have a lot of peer volunteers who work with us in veterans justice outreach who work with people who are involved in the criminal system, which is a place you find a lot of people who will not go to a doctor, but end up funneling down into the Nation's largest mental health system, our prisons and jails. And VA has become an incredibly active partner in reaching that population, largely through peers.

Mr. Zeldin. And I do understand that your peer specialists do a lot, and more so than I would have list obviously, because you are intimately familiar with it. But I do understand that your peer specialists do a lot of that. But I am getting feedback that there aren't as many peer support groups as necessary.

Dr. Kudler. I think you are right. And I think VA can be in many ways the hub that can help generate more peer support. The Clay Hunt Act asked us to partner with community peer programs where they existed, and we are doing that and following the Clay Hunt Act in trying to enlarge on what Clay Hunt asked for.

But I think we could be doing more. We have developed a peer support specialist training that, I think we could be sharing with other groups. And I would like to see that happen. I think particularly for Guard and Reserve. I have been in Suffolk County. I am from Queens. But I have worked with military members and reserve units there, and I think that peer support could be key in dealing with them.

Mr. Zeldin. Yeah. Peer support is important. I had real training in the peer support groups. In Suffolk County we are one of over a dozen counties in New York State, we have something called the PFC Joseph Dwyer Program. We will put 8, 10, 12 veterans in one room because people feel isolated and alone. They don't realize that someone around the block is going through what they are going through. So it is tearing apart families. People at work may not understand. Friends don't understand. So it is very important to create that peer group setting.

Also a lot of people may live at a distance from a VA hospital, so having support groups out in the community is incredibly important. One of the things that I have noticed while serving on this

Committee, we have had many representatives from the VA come before this Committee.

I have only been on—this is my first term in Congress. I have only been able to experience this a little over year. A lot of the opening statements that we hear from the VA representatives are telling the Committee about everything that is working, to create this picture of the VA as if it is perfect. And we all know it is not. And what was stated by Dr. McCarthy was, I want to be transparent, "want to be transparent."

And what we hear from our constituents with regard to veteran crisis line, calling a patient advocate and getting a voicemail, in some cases not getting a call back. The Denver VA hospital construction project last year there was a last minute bailout where obviously the fiscal situation could have been brought to this Committee's attention earlier, a backlog of appeals where a backlog of claims is reduced, just creating a backlog of appeals.

We hear constituents with individual cases where their ducks are lined up, paperwork is in order and they are still waiting. We read the USA Today report a few weeks ago where supervisors are instructing employees to falsify wait time lists. I would just—one observation from one freshman members of this particular Committee, I think in the effort of wanting to be transparent, it would be very helpful if when you were coming to the Committee right out of the gate you are telling us what needs to be fixed as opposed to this Committee having it to pull out of you. I yield back.

The CHAIRMAN. Mr. McNerney?

Mr. MCNERNEY. I thank the Chairman. This is a difficult and humbling subject, so I tread on it carefully. I am going to ask—I am going to direct most of my questions to you, Dr. Maffucci. But I ask anyone else on the panel to jump in if they have answers. Dr. Maffucci, you referred to the Clay Hunt Save Act as a step in the right direction. What specifically in that law is working that we can expand upon?

Dr. MAFFUCCI. So as I alluded to in my testimony, this year has really been the foundation. We have been—the VSO community has been included in conversations with VA about how do we do this right, because it is one thing to do it, but it is—and our intention was always not to just get a law passed, it was to make sure that it was implemented correctly.

So I think certainly going through the evaluations process, I previously worked in the Pentagon, worked for DoD and I was on the Army's Suicide Prevention Task Force for about two and a half years. And the Army went through this. And it took them a good three or four years to kind of process, figure out how to go through evaluating their mental health programs. It is something that is not done within the mental health worlds. There are no standards that are required. There are no metrics that are standardized. And so it makes these kinds of program evaluations really challenging. But our vision for the Clay Hunt Save Act was that to ask the VA to step up and set those standards and work with DoD to do that, because DoD has those same requirements.

So I am really, I think we are really excited about the evaluations piece. Certainly with the loan repayment program for psychiatrists, we were hoping that that would get implemented more quickly. I understand there has been some challenges with changing the law basically to allow that. But I think that too, noting that one of the challenges to VA hiring is the low salaries. The more that the VA can provide those incentives and can match the private sector, if you will, the more competitive they can be to bring in those professionals. So that was another piece that we are really excited about.

And then certainly the partnerships. Up until recently, up until Secretary McDonald came into leadership at VA, partnerships was not a word that the VA uttered. And so that in and of itself over the last two years is immense. And we hope to see that term and the implementation of what that term is, we are really working to make sure that those partnerships expand in a really innovative way.

We have seen a lot of really positive interaction between VA, IAVA, the others at this table. It is going to take time. And unfortunately that is just the way it is. But I think we all feel, if I can speak for the others on the panel, we all feel that we are moving in the right direction, that the momentum is there, the motivation is there. There is a different energy and we are doing this. Like I said in my testimony, we have stopped talking about it, we are actually doing things.

Mr. ZELDIN. Well, one of the things we—the buzzwords these days is evidence-based. And, of course, suicide it is very difficult to get sort of trials or anything like that. But data sharing can be extremely important, not only in this issue, but with regard to post-traumatic stress and traumatic brain injuries. What are the obstacles we are facing with regard to data sharing, anyone on the panel?

Dr. MAFFUCCI. So one of the challenges, which as a taxpayer doesn't make sense to me, is that most of the data that is paid for with taxpayer dollars is not shared. This is actually, I believe I heard Dr. Shulkin commit the VA to actually opening up the VA's vaults. And in sharing that, they figure out how to make sure that the data that the VA holds is shared across the research community. These are dollars that have already—the taxpayers have already put forward to get that research, to get that data. And I can—I promise you that there are other researchers out there that are just chomping at the bit to get at it and to help and to do their part.

Mr. ZELDIN. Are the HIPAA laws part of the—

Dr. MAFFUCCI. I think that is part of the concern is the HIPAA. And how do you go—how do you balance needing to know certain information with also protecting the patient's identity. So that is certainly a challenge. But I would also say in my own personal opinion I think there is—HIPAA is often called upon as like the scary elephant in the room, right.

Mr. ZELDIN. Right.

Dr. MAFFUCCI. When people want to—when people are worried about data sharing for whatever reason, often HIPAA is the primary reason put forward. And the law itself often gets interpreted wrong.

Mr. ZELDIN. Mr. Chairman, perhaps we could assemble a group of experts to decide how to use data sharing and not violate HIPAA intent.

The CHAIRMAN. Absolutely, great idea.

Mr. ZELDIN. I yield back.

The CHAIRMAN. I appreciate it. Ms. Radewagen, do you have any comments?

Ms. RADEWAGEN. Thank you, Mr. Chairman. First of all, all of this information has been tremendously useful and I want to thank you all for being here today. I also wanted to associate myself with Mr. Coffman and Ms. Rice's concerns about the other than honorable discharged veterans. We do have a couple of cases back in my home district about that. And one veteran is in such bad shape his heart has become enlarged. He was in Afghanistan and Iraq and he was court martialed. So we are trying to work some kind of things out. I also have a brother who is a disabled veteran from Vietnam, he has got mental health problems big time. And VA prescribes tons and tons of pills. And so I understand the importance of it.

But I have a quick question for Ms. Ruocco. And it has to do with family and survival involvement. Do you think VA does a sufficient job supporting the surviving family members of veterans who have died by suicide? And if not, how can VA improve in that area? There are all these problems that the veterans are going through, their families are going through the same thing.

Ms. RUOCCO. Right. Actually, in the past, you know, as far as TAPS, our mission statement was mostly focused on active duty servicemembers who died by suicide. But we have just expanded that and we are just working on a memorandum of understanding with the VA to bring in surviving families right to the tragedy assistance program for survivors where we can provide them, you know, very comprehensive care right from day one and get them, you know, feel—getting the kind of care they need, peer support as far—and also connected to trauma support, counseling, you know, any kind of benefits issues, anything like that. So, yes, we are moving in a direction where we are doing better about that.

What we hear from our families is they would like to be more involved before there is a death, and because they feel like they are at home struggling with veterans that are very sick and just don't know how to get them into treatment, don't know how to convince them to go to the VA, don't know how to, you know, where to go to ask for advice, where to get support for that. So I think there is a real need for the VA to work closer with families on providing them access to professionals who can guide them and peers who can support the process.

Ms. RADEWAGEN. Thank you, Mr. Chairman. I yield back.

The CHAIRMAN. Thank you very much. Dr. Abraham, you're recognized.

Mr. ABRAHAM. Thank you, Mr. Chairman. This is a most important hearing. I thank you for having it. When I was fortunate enough to be put on this Committee about a year and a half ago, the first day we were told that 22 veterans were committing suicide and that if 17 of those could get into the VA system then we could certainly reduce that. And we hear these same numbers today. And you feel the frustration up here on the dais and I am sure in your arena too. The frustration is palpable because we understand that, yeah, we are dealing with a bureaucracy, but come on, we have got to do better than this, because when we—like you said, Dr. Maffucci—we need more assessment and we need planning.

But I guarantee if I gave you guys at the table right now a legal pad and a pencil, in two hours you could come up with a plan, you know how to fix this. And I know that this probably goes above your level as to the implementation and the move, but it is not like we are dealing with bronchitis here. We are dealing with lives every day.

Somebody, I think it was Mr. Huelskamp, brought up the Choice Program. I have got physicians that in my district, in my state that have tried to get into the VA system. They are just dead in the water literally as far as getting movement. And these are physicians that are in good standing with their state medical boards, they graduated from accredited universities and they have no criminal activity. And that is all you need. And you can do that in a matter of 30 seconds on a computer now to bring these people in and get some help in the community, because I know the VA and the DoD is overwhelmed.

And, Dr. Berger, you mentioned that DoD and VA are not still talking to each other on electronic health matters. And if they duplicate a medicine from one doctor to another or if they give them medicine that has an intersection, yeah, you have got some very serious problems very quicky.

Our Chairman made a comment that, you know, why a pilot program when we are talking about this phone system? We know the Secretary and certainly his supervisors under him have the ability to move manpower to wherever that need is. So why do we need a study to study a study and why do we need a pilot program? Let's try something, because what we have tried since I have been here hasn't been too sporting. And we are dealing with people's lives every day.

So, again, you know, the frustration, we need to quit talking and we need to do something productive here. Ms. Radewagen mentioned the families. And I would say, well, we talk about HIPAA, you know, that big elephant in the room that you can't, you know, share what size clothes you wear that day with somebody. When that veteran comes in, because I have run medical practices all my life and, you know, I understand HIPAA compliance, but I also understand HIPAA what it takes to put that name on a form. If you explain to that veteran when they come in what—whoever they list on the HIPAA form can access their information, they could have in 90 times out of 100 they are going to say put them on the list. Call them.

And we know there is four physicians down here, five physicians up here. Those on the dais that aren't physicians, I guarantee you they are more intelligent than I am, that they—we understand that family is the first person or the first unit that recognizes when this veteran is in a bind. These are the ones that can reach out. And we have got to incorporate them. You guys have got to get them in the VA system better so that they can help. And when they do see an instance they can call and not get a recording. And again, just comments, I will take any, you know, comments you have. Ms. Ruocco?

Ms. RUOCCO. Yes, thank you for that. That is really important. One of the things that we worry about is that, you know, all my families told me that they wish they would have had evidence-based treatment for the injuries and illnesses that they had. And so, yes, while the Clay Hunt Act has incentives for psychiatrists, psychiatrists give medication. They don't do evidence-based treatment for PTSD. So we have got to get the time and the providers to give the treatment that these guys need, these men and women that are coming back with these kinds of injuries. We have to have the time, the space, and the professionals, you know, middle level mental health providers that are actually doing treatment and we have got to have incentives for that as well.

Mr. ABRAHAM. Thank you. Dr. Berger, do you have any comment?

Dr. BERGER. I think my colleague, Kim, is right on with it. But I would also like to say that I think there needs to be more effort at coordination. This is a national public health problem and veterans are a big part of it and we can focus on that. But what is important is the VA needs to take the leadership role in this, in coordinating this. They have got practices, they have got standards, et cetera. Do it. I know it is going to burden Harold's shop and Dr. McCarthy's shop. Let's find the money so that we can bolster the resources there to do it. Let's do it.

Mr. ABRAHAM. Thank you, Chairman. I yield back.

The CHAIRMAN. Dr. Wenstrup?

Mr. WENSTRUP. Thank you, Mr. Chairman. I appreciate you all being here today. I found it interesting today when you talked about that number 22. And we have heard that over and over and over again. And with my limited psychology background, which is an undergraduate degree, negativity over and over again is not helping in this situation. Created awareness, which was very much needed, but it doesn't help. And I hope we take a turn in the other direction, not only VA, but in the public in general. And I also found it intriguing and hopeful that as more people get into care the rate drops and that is the bottom line.

Another interesting point is it is not really just being deployed, it is the non-deployed. And what you just mentioned, Dr. Berger, has been weighing on my mind all along, because just in my neighborhood where I grew up, middle class, upper middle class, three families have had suicides, they went to good schools. You know, the things that you would think would be the underlying factors they committed suicide. So it is not just in the military. Now, as you said, the military can lead on this with the opportunity to do that. But this is more than that.

You mentioned the HIPAA restrictions, if you will. And Dr. Tim Murphy, who is a Navy veteran, psychologist, Member of Congress, has a very good bill, I believe. It is out and I would encourage you to take a look at it and weigh in on it from the standpoint of being able to engage the family more readily. And I think that will help us not only at the VA, but also in society.

So, you know, you don't see many suicides taking place in theater, they happen after. You know, my feeling as a veteran when you are in theater you are engaged, you are a part of something big, you are important, you have a purposes. And I think that when that purpose is taken away and you find yourself with nothing to do, that is when you become more vulnerable. We have put a lot of it on, oh, you were in combat. But we are seeing you weren't in combat. So did we predetermine the cause erroneously and now we are starting to get it? Is it important that we get people involved with part of something positive? And that is probably the case on the civilian side too. So I would love for you to weigh in on those thoughts. And I really appreciate you all being here today.

Dr. MCCARTHY. So could I just start? I so appreciate what you said, Dr. Wenstrup. I think you are 100 percent on target. What I was trying to communicate earlier is we need to approach it in the same way we approach preventing heart disease. You know, it is not like it starts in the ICU that we focus on prevention. And the same is true, it doesn't start with our crisis line and it doesn't start in that urgent situation all the time. Sometimes it does. But we really need to take the steps ahead of time. And it is not just for veterans and not just for military, but it is for everybody.

And increasing awareness is really important and making it a discussable issue is also really important, because the loneliness that comes from the stigma and the fear about getting treatment is a big piece of it. So we agree with you and we are happy to work—we have partnered with other Federal agencies, SAMHSA and CMS and so forth also to address this, because it is a national crisis. It is not just veterans, but it is veterans included.

Dr. KUDLER. May I add if I might? Just yesterday at the Invictus Games, which were mentioned earlier, it was announced that VA is partnering with Give an Hour and their Change Direction Program. Prince Harry also made a video about Change Direction. The idea is to develop basic mental health literacy for all Americans. It is not surprising that veterans like all Americans don't have words for their feelings and don't know where to go when they have a mental health problem, and don't know if they should even speak about it, since obviously nobody else speaks about it. So we are partnering to create a national rollout of a mental health literacy program, which we believe will help this generation and future generations, not just veterans, but all Americans.

Dr. MCCARTHY. And I would just like to add to that. With the repeated number of times from various people on the panel spoke about the peer programs, whether that is the necessity for peer family connections, as well as that veteran connection, and not just being in the VA, but expanding that program that works so well in the VA out into the community, into the chat rooms, you know, into the various places where veterans are in colleges and, you know, other locations so that they can bring them in, because you can have the best system in the world and the greatest programs and services, but if you can't get them there, if they don't feel, you know, why is it important and understand the treatment works, you know, you have lost right at the beginning.

Ms. RUOCCO. Right. We know that, you know, it is a sense of purpose and a sense of belongingness are protective factors for suicide. And so, you know, that is one of the big losses that the military have when they get out and go into the communities and they struggle. Where do I belong? What is my purpose in life? So these peer groups within the communities are really important. At TAPS we have good grief camps at every one of our national events. And we match active duty military or veterans with a child who has lost a parent or a sibling to suicide or other deaths in the military. Out of that comes a new sense of purpose where I can mentor this child of a fallen comrade, right.

And they also find a new sense of belongingness with other mentors, where we keep them connected with one another. And so out of those pages and connecting them we see people become at risk, but they are connected to other people, they have a place where people notice that and connect them with care. And so building those kinds of things all over the country is what is going to help support what the VA is doing.

Mr. WENSTRUP. Prevention is always wonderful if we can do it. And I think we are getting some signs on what will work. Dr. Berger?

Dr. BERGER. You have already heard my comments about VA taking a leadership role. But in a larger sense, and it maybe shows my scientific nerdiness, you can't manage what you don't measure. And so just a number of people passing through a program does not tell you whether the program works or not.

Mr. WENSTRUP. Agreed.

Dr. BERGER. So—

Mr. WENSTRUP. Yes.

Dr. MAFFUCCI. So I just wanted to add from our own members survey we know that our members, so 80 percent, over 80 percent have told us that they have experienced transitioning challenges. And the top three challenges that have been identified, number one is loss of identity or purposes. Two is finding or keeping employment. And we actually know from our survey that for those who took part, 65 percent did not have a job when they left the military, so again tying back into a loss of purpose. Jobs often give us purpose. Careers give us purpose. And then finally the third one was mental health concerns.

So we do know within our population some of the pieces, or at least within our membership, some of the pieces that are challenging within transition. And it is a start: the peer support programs, getting individuals connected while they are still on base. The installation access last year was huge for DoD to allow these programs and partnerships to come on base. One of the things that DoD has not provided and I don't believe is tracking from my inquiries is how that is being utilized: what installations, who is coming to the installations, what does that look like? And that would be really important too to understand how you connect people to RWB, to Rubicon, to the organizations here before they even leave that installation.

Mr. WENSTRUP. Well, thank you. My time is expired. I appreciate it.

The CHAIRMAN. Thank you very much. Final questions from the Ranking Member, Ms. Brown.

Ms. BROWN. Thank you, Mr. Chairman. And this has been a very informative session. I have got to thank you very, very much, very educational. And I want to make a couple of comments and then I want to turn it over to you to answer some questions that I didn't really hear the answers to. First, My VA 12 breakthrough priorities. I think that's wonderful. But it should be something on top of it as far as I am concerned pertaining to suicides, because that is—when we tackle homelessness, when we were able to engage the mayors and the community and the VA took the lead, I mean we brought that down. And I think we can do the same with VA as the leadership.

And so the veterans crisis hotline have come under scrutiny, have had some problems. It has been realigned. And I met with the team and I felt that they are on the right track. The vet centers, everybody knows they do an excellent job. Those, you should have the peers in all of the vet centers in my opinion, the peer to peer and then the training of the VA counsel suicide is different from that peer to peer. But the vet centers is to me in the community and they do an excellent job.

I haven't heard enough about the female veterans. I have had several forums with them. They have said, and we are coming up with the Women's Veterans Memorial that we go every year. But they are not educated to what services are available. I don't understand why the women get such a fallout. But they don't know what services are available and they don't really view them as a part of when they get out as a part of the system. So we really need to do some work in that area.

And I do want to hear about the Vietnam veterans, because when I went to this conference, that is the one area that stood out saying that the Vietnam veterans are one of the highest groups committing suicide, because when they came back they didn't feel integrated, appreciated. And so we need some special reach out for them.

And the last thing I want to mention is as we—one way to get additional professionals is to work with the colleges and give scholarships in that area. And to me that is the key, to give those scholarships, not just for psychiatrists, but social works and other areas. Everybody don't have to be a doctor to give assistance. And, of course, I—you know, to get assistance that maybe you need a doctor, but some of us may need the entry level to be referred to a doctor. So with that I want to hear from everybody.

Dr. MCCARTHY. So I will start on this end and then we will keep going. We have gotten very loud and clear the message about the 12 priorities, so thank you for communicating that very effectively. We agree the crisis line has been reorganized. And we are really pleased that there will be a total of 343 responders employed by the crisis line. We definitely feel like that is moving in the right direction. And the alliance of that group is in the right place.

Thanks for celebrating our vet centers. We are very proud of them and they are very key partners for all of us. Regarding women vets, we need to do better. We need to have a welcoming environment. We need—we have heard from them what sometimes is perceived as less than welcoming. We need to fix what that is. But in addition, we welcome all the help in getting the word out about VA is there for them. We have a communications campaign, I Serve Too, VA is there for you too. You know, we have done a lot with images and so forth to include women veterans, but it is not enough. We also are looking at how inclusive we are in treatment programs and research studies and everything else.

The Vietnam vets, the Secretary rolled out a 50-year celebration campaign. And we have been awarding a number of vets welcome home medals recognizing their 50 years of service, including some of our own employees who teared up in ways I have never seen. It has taken us way too long to say welcome home as a Nation. And, you know, we do that individually, but to have the 50-year anniversary be a reason to do it has been a really important thing.

We agree with you about colleges and scholarships. I will pass this to the rest of the panel.

Ms. RUOCCO. Hi. Thank you so much. You know, one thing I hear from the families all the time is that they worry how their loved one died will kind of be what people focus on and they will forget how they lived and served. Many of our families and in my testimony there are some stories of those families where they went into the military and they were healthy and strong. They did several tours and it wasn't until after they had that exposure and that trauma that they started to get in trouble and having drinking and other issues that then got them less than honorable discharges or other things. So we really have got to look at, you know, what are we asking these human beings to do? Let's provide them the kind of mental health care that they deserve after all these exposures.

Another challenge that we have had is the vet centers are awesome and they do really good counseling for our family members. But you have to have been in a combat zone to go to the vet center. So where there, once again, is another fall through the cracks. If we have a servicemembers, and we know in the active duty 50 percent of the people who die by suicide have never been in combat. They are struggling with other things and they may have been held back from combat because of their struggles. They are not eligible for vet center care. So we have got to look at those people who don't fit into those things and really fill in those gaps as well. Thank you.

Dr. BERGER. Thank you, Congresswoman, for your questions and your comments related to Vietnam vets, so I will limit my comments to them, to us. As you know, back in March the Secretary issued or the VA publically announced nine initiatives to deal with suicide. And one of those, I quote the VA itself "Using predictive modeling to guide early interventions for suicide prevention." They need, as I said earlier, to develop a nationwide strategy to address the problems of suicides among our older veterans. As I said earlier, there are many risk factors that we share with our younger colleagues, but what is it that sets us apart and makes us take our lives more frequently, according to the 2013 data.

Ms. ILEM. I would just comment that VA has made tremendous progress on women veterans issues and attention from the committee on women veteran's issues. A number of hearings have been held, bills have been introduced. And I think one of the things that is borne out by the research that VA has done on women veterans is that once you get them in the VA they are doing, you know, much better off. They are much better off, they are getting the services that they need. But it is addressing that issue of how do you get those from other military eras? We know that VA did a tremendous outreach program for Operation Enduring Freedom/Operation Iraqi Freedom veterans. And it resulted in a much higher rate of those veterans coming in and being seen and be part of the system. But how do we get those other eras of veterans, women veterans, who have felt neglected, have felt isolated and could really benefit from VA services? So I think an outreach program to them, specifically targeted based on just what has been successful in VA, would be a really—would be tremendous for those people.

Dr. MAFFUCCI. So IAVA has been preparing to really roll out our campaign focused around women veterans. Last year our research department did an eight-city tour meeting with some of our women veteran members, as well as a survey that were sent out beyond our membership to really kind of try to understand what the challenges are. From myself my first question was are the challenges that women veterans face different from their male compatriots or are they the same? And if they are the same then what do we do if they are different, what do we do? And I think one of the women that I spoke with in one of the focus groups summed it up the best, where she said, "Our challenges are the same, but the resources aren't tailored to women and the women veterans are having challenges finding the resources."

A few things that I really pulled out from the survey findings and from those conversations that I wanted to share, our members, our women veterans they self-identify. They are proud to be veterans. But they are also tired of defending the fact that they are veterans to the Nation at large. Being asked, being challenged and then when they come out and they tell people that they are veterans, and having a look of disbelief or a question. All right, this is a cultural change first and foremost. And it is a cultural change not just at VA, it is the Nation. We all need to recognize that women are growing in the forces, they are growing in the veteran community, they are serving and they are serving right next to the men that are enlisting as well.

On the topic of peer support, that was something that our survey showed women really want other women in peer support programs. It is a concern that we have had just looking across the peer support program that already exists and understanding are minority groups represented, to what degree, are we making sure that the populations that peers are available to peers? This is something that we are going to keep working on, because it is so critical, both within VA, but also outside of VA to create that network of peer support so that women can find other women, share their stories and know they are not alone.

The other piece is just the research piece is critical. And it is not just VA. Across the Federal agencies there is not a requirement to look at programs and look at gender analysis and look at age analysis and look at some of the other covariants that occur when you want to understand a program is working. It is past time that the Federal agencies at large start to recognize it is not just about that big picture. We have got to start understanding the populations within the population at large.

The CHAIRMAN. Thank you very much, Members. Thank you to our panelists for being here today. I would ask that unanimous consent that all Members will have five legislative days with which to revise and extend their remarks and add any extraneous material. And with that this hearing is adjourned.

[Whereupon, at 12:28 p.m., the Committee was adjourned.]

# APPENDIX

## Prepared Statement of Corrine Brown, Ranking Member

Thank you, Mr. Chairman, for calling this hearing today.

Strong oversight of the Department's Suicide Prevention Programs remains a priority of this Committee. We are all aware of the often cited statistic of 22 veterans a day committing suicide.

We also know that VA reported in 2014 that there is decreased rates of suicide among users of the Veterans Health Care System with mental health conditions.

The question becomes how do we ensure ready access to safe, quality, mental health services for veterans in need of care?

I hope the VA witnesses here today will be able to update us on these numbers, as much of the country was not included in previous estimates.

One subject that concerns me relates to the new MyVA 12 breakthrough priorities. I understand that addressing the suicide problem is not one of them. 'Increase access to healthcare', 'improve the compensation and pension exam', 'continue to reduce homelessness' and 'transform the supply chain' are all on the list, but specifically reducing suicide is not included. Given that suicide, nationally, is considered by some to be a public health problem, I believe VA should include suicide prevention as one of their MyVA priorities.

I look forward to VA's testimony on this and where suicide prevention fits into the 12 priorities. I know that the urgency of this issue is not lost upon the VA. VA leads the nation in service related mental health treatment, and rightfully so.

The Suicide Data Report of 2012 was published by the VA partially as a result of the 2007 Joshua Omvig (AHM-vig) Veterans Suicide Prevention Act. This law was a positive first step in addressing what was then a burgeoning epidemic of suicides in the veteran community. It required, among other things, the VA to establish a comprehensive program for suicide prevention among veterans. Additionally, it required the creation of a suicide prevention counselor at each VA medical facility, who are responsible to engage in outreach to veterans. Finally, this law required VA to set up a toll-free hotline.

Mr. Chairman, this hearing will also examine the implementation of the Clay Hunt Suicide Prevention for American Veterans Act. Passed in the early days of the 114th Congress, this law focused the nation on this terrible epidemic affecting veterans of the current cohort.

This law requires the Secretary of Veterans Affairs and the Secretary of Defense to arrange for an outside evaluation of their mental health care and suicide prevention programs.

It also requires any service member being discharged to have their case reviewed for any evidence of Post-Traumatic Stress Disorder or Traumatic Brain Injury or Military Sexual Trauma.

We have been at war for over 14 years. There are many veterans out there who do not engage the VA health care system for purposes of mental health treatment, veterans from all eras. Today, the discussion should include how VA is going to reach these veterans, what better ways can be used to ensure access to quality mental health care, and finally, once veterans are engaged, how do we keep them engaged. It is time to think outside the box and tackle this very pervasive problem.

Thank you, Mr. Chairman and I yield back the balance of my time.

---

## Prepared Statement of Tim Walz

I think these two articles are especially pertinent in light of the discussion we are having today in the committee. As a community, as a nation, and as members of the House Committee on Veterans Affairs, we need to fully understand the occurrence of clustering in units and work to prevent these deaths. I look forward to fur-

48

ther discussion on the ways we can reach Veterans who are not receiving the care and benefits they have earned and deserve.

### Suicide hits hard among the ranks of Minnesota National Guard

A father's despair over his son's death in Iraq drives home a suicide crisis for Minnesota National Guard.
**By Mark Brunswick Star Tribune**

APRIL 2, 2016 - 7:48AM

Kim Schmit knew her husband was in trouble, that much was clear.

It had been seven years since the Willmar couple's 26-year-old son, Josh, had been killed by a roadside bomb in Iraq while serving in the Army. Greg Schmit, an 18-year member of the Minnesota National Guard, had found it particularly hard to adjust.

Out of guilt and grief, his life had dissolved into a series of unproductive counseling sessions at the VA. A medley of medications for anxiety, depression and sleeplessness now frequently left him either lethargic or irritable. Contributing to his despair, he contended that the Guard had been unsupportive after Josh's death and that a few commanders had conspired to ruin his career and have him fired.

Late on a July night last year, Kim would later tell authorities, she was awakened by her husband struggling for breath next to her. She spotted the prescription bottles. All were empty. Within minutes, Greg Schmit, the by-the-book supply sergeant, was rushed to the hospital in a futile attempt to save his life.

"I tried with Greg," Kim Schmit said, "but I wasn't enough to keep him going."

Few organizations have felt the crisis in military suicides more than the Minnesota National Guard. In the past five years, more of its members have died by suicide than all but one state Guard in the country. Minnesota's Guard is the 10th largest state Guard by size. But when it comes to suicide, its 27 deaths rank second only to Pennsylvania's 30.

By comparison, the state of Minnesota overall ranks 41st in the country in the rate of suicides per 100,000 people.

Asked if the Minnesota Guard has a suicide problem, Command Sgt. Major Douglas Wortham, the Guard's top enlisted soldier, said simply: "One life lost to suicide is too many."

Guard leaders say they can't explain why only the Pennsylvania Guard has recorded more suicides. Stressors in everyday life - job loss, financial difficulties, relationship and mental health issues and substance abuse - more than Guard service are likely contributing factors, they say.

"We see our soldiers two days out of the month, but the community, the churches, their employers, they get to see them those other 28 days out of the month," said Maj Ron Jarvi, program manager for the Minnesota National Guard Resilience Risk Reduction & Suicide Prevention Office.

Changes in record keeping - Guard units did not keep uniform records on suicides until recently - could also account for the high number. So, too, could a possible "contagion" effect, where suicide might be considered more acceptable the more it happens around you.

"With each suicide you have an increased pool risk of suicide," said Melissa Heinen, suicide prevention coordinator for the Minnesota Department of Health, who has worked closely with the Guard. "The more suicides you have, the more that becomes a more normalized option."

### The new reality

On a snowy Friday morning, more than 70 soldiers file into a classroom at the Minnesota National Guard Armory in Cottage Grove. At first it seems like just another meeting during just another drill weekend.

But as Capt. Tony Hodgkins takes the podium, it quickly becomes clear it is about something deeper. Hodgkins, the unit commander, asks the soldiers how many have experienced someone close to them feeling suicidal. Nearly half raise their hands.

This is the new reality of the National Guard, where suicide prevention has become not only a priority, but a necessity. In the last eight years, Hodgkins tells the group, about 40 members of the Minnesota Guard have taken their lives.

Most have been men. The average age of victims was 26 - much younger than the middle-aged males in the general population who kill themselves. The most common cause of death - a self-inflicted gunshot.

Some, such as the 41-year-old Guard member who shot himself while sheriff's deputies pleaded with him, had been deployed, police reports and other documents show. But fewer than half - 17 of 41 - had been deployed or seen combat experience.

In 2015, a 27-year-old full-time member of the Honor Guard at Fort Snelling who had never been deployed killed himself in his apartment within two weeks of being told he was failing Officer Candidate School. The year before, a 21-year-old Guardsman killed himself after drinking heavily and arguing with friends. He died 10 days after joining the Guard and before he was scheduled to ship out to boot camp.

In an effort to address the issue, the Guard has taken steps in recent years to ensure that each Minnesota unit has a resilience leader trained to identify common stressors and recommend resources. Each unit also has scheduled an annual block of suicide prevention training that includes role-playing and videos.

The Guard also is employing new techniques and technologies - using Internet resources and social media connections - to reach out to soldiers.

"We live by soldier's creed and warrior's ethos and after it's all said and done and we stand at attention and declare these things we've memorized, it really just means we're here for each other," Hodgkins tells the group. "At least we're supposed to be."

On this winter morning, soldiers are assigned to the 204th Area Medical Support Co., whose mission is to provide health support to Army units wherever they are deployed, including the battlefield. Staff Sgt. Mandie McGinnis, one of the unit's suicide intervention officers, takes the lead.

"I want you to take your masks off if you are having a bad day," she urges the class. "Somebody can help talk you through it and find the light at the other side."

Leaders hand out cards outlining suicide risk factors, along with a card listing suicide-prevention hot line numbers. Each soldier is given a gun lock. McGinnis also leads a role-playing session where she steps on a table and pretends to be thinking about jumping off a bridge. Several soldiers in the class volunteer to step forward to talk her out of it.

McGinnis, whose regular Guard job is in medical supply, and several other unit members recently started a Facebook page to help soldiers in need. It is a resource for nearly any type of support. The page, Battle Check, is available only to current and former service members. As evidence that it is filling a need, it now has more than 2,500 members nationwide. As the Friday morning session winds down, 1st Sgt. Brent Ambuehl, the senior enlisted member of the unit, addresses the group.

"The scariest thing for me as part of a command team is suicide," he says. "That's the 11th-hour call that I fear the most. Losing a soldier in your ranks to something that is this preventable is plain-out scary. This is a group effort here and we all need to take care of each other."

### 'Pins and needles'

Even with all the Guard's prevention efforts, the death last summer of Greg Schmit illustrates the stark difference between how things work in training and what actually plays out in real life.

In response to Schmit's death, the Guard told the Star Tribune that it ensured that he had access to mental health, family survivor specialists and spiritual counseling; and that his behavior - even before his son's death - was "inconsistent with standards of military order and discipline."

But his wife and others believe the Guard's treatment of Schmit after his son was killed contributed to his grief and ultimately, his death. Five years before Schmit took his life, after a series of increasingly tense workplace confrontations and accusations of disrespect and insubordination, his commanders had fired him from his full-time job as a supply sergeant at the Willmar armory.

"It reminded me of a soldier who was injured laying on the battlefield and they were stepping over him, letting him bleed out," Kim Schmit said recently.

As the Guard moved closer to firing him, it sought insight about his behavior from the soldiers he worked with. More than a dozen wrote letters of support. But several claimed Schmit used Josh's death as an excuse for behavior they described as unsettling.

One first sergeant wrote that Schmit, who had made some enemies, had been told many times before and after his son's death, "to change his behavior," according to paperwork Kim Schmit provided to the Star Tribune. "Now when he is told to change his behavior, his response is how people are out to get him because his son died."

Another complained of walking on "pins and needles" on the anniversary of Josh's death, and of feeling threatened because Schmit had access to weapons.

One supportive soldier wrote that many people felt Schmit "needs to get over it and move on with his life" and were "getting sick of him using his son's death as an excuse to have an outburst." Yet, he added, others recognized Schmit "will never get over the loss of his son, and he has the right to grieve his son."

In November 2010, the Guard cited seven incidents over the previous two years in which Schmit was accused of disrespect, insubordination or failure to obey orders, including a 2009 letter of reprimand in which he was docked three days' pay. It also listed four incidents before Josh's death to show what it called "the prolonged and continued nature of your anger problems."

A month later, Schmit made a passionate plea to stay in the Guard and "continue to serve my country, bring stability to my family, and honor the values and way of life (of) Joshua, and many like him, who paid the ultimate sacrifice to protect."

The following March, Major Gen. Richard Nash, head of the Minnesota Guard, signed the letter dismissing Schmit. The letter, officially called an "Involuntary Separation Care Plan," offered the names of resources for support.

"I encourage you to take advantage of these resources to assist you through this difficult time," Nash's letter said.

That same month, Schmit attempted suicide for the first time. He would tell doctors that he remembered waking up after taking an overdose of pills and being angry that he had survived.

Asked about how it felt it responded to the situation, the Guard said in a recent written response: "After Sgt. Joshua Schmit's death - even with sympathetic and caring leaders and full access to counseling - Staff Sgt. Greg Schmit continued his behavior, resulting in progressive nonjudicial punishment and ultimately termination of his employment."

Veterans advocate Trisha Appeldorn, director of the Kandiyohi County Veterans Services Office and an acquaintance of the Schmits, learned about Greg Schmit's struggle after he asked her to help him fill out paperwork. She said she was stunned by how he was treated.

"Anyone would be shocked," she said. "A father loses his son in Iraq and basically gets booted out of the National Guard two years before he could retire. In my opinion, it was just sort of a raw deal."

### Emotionally 'stuck'

After being dismissed from the Guard, Schmit's condition worsened. He was treated briefly at a hospital in Pueblo, Colo., then entered the Warrior Transition Battalion at Fort Riley, Kansas. It was one of several programs set up by the Army to help wounded soldiers transition back into the military or to civilian life.

He was medically discharged from the Army in 2013 due to headaches, depression and post-traumatic stress.

More than 1,000 pages of notes from the Minneapolis and St. Cloud VAs that Kim Schmit obtained document his slide. The reports are dominated by words such as "resentment," "unresolved anger," and "hopelessness."

Greg Schmit told of having vivid word-for-word conversations with Josh in his dreams, described flashbacks of seeing his son's dead body and discussed the once-a-week panic attacks that put pain in his chest and blinded his eyes.

lot" of distress, and he experiences feelings of worthlessness. He reported that he has unpleasant dreams about these two situations every night. He described the dreams as "very vivid." He stated that he has "word for word" conversations with his son in the dreams. He described another dream as "being on trial" for his work-related issues. He indicated that the dreams cause him "a lot" of distress. He endorsed experiencing flashbacks every day, saying that "everything comes back to his mind." He described the flashbacks as the "reoccurrence of his work situation" and his "son's crispy body." He described being confused and "blanking out" for 10-15 minutes. He endorsed experiencing emotional reactivity every day. He gets upset and experiences "mild" panic symptoms when people do not listen to what he is saying. He described having a physical reaction in which he has a pain in his chest and "blinders coming across my eyes." This happens once per week. His reaction lasts

An excerpt from Gregory Schmit's VA patient file.

In one meeting with a VA staff psychiatrist, Schmit admitted that he was emotionally "stuck." In a 2013 session for medication management and supportive therapy, he spoke of having regular nightmares and feelings of worthlessness. He also told the doctor he would attempt suicide if he knew it wouldn't hurt other people.

51

Two years later, after more counseling failed to help, Greg Schmit killed himself. The cause of death was listed as intentional multiple drug overdose, with a secondary cause listed as major depression and post-traumatic stress disorder. He was 56.

Schmit was buried alongside his son at Fairview Cemetery in Willmar. Because he had been fired, the Guard no longer considered him a member at the time of his death. Nor does it consider Schmit to be one of its suicide victims.

"The circumstances surrounding the Schmit family are tragic," the Guard said recently, when asked to respond to his death, adding that its "thoughts and prayers . are with the Schmit family."

Kim Schmit, meanwhile, has been left to shoulder the deaths of two soldiers: a son killed just 10 days before he was to come home and a husband who blamed himself for the loss. She said her son, like his father, "wanted to play the Army game." Greg encouraged Josh to enlist and when Josh died, Greg "thought he killed his son in a roundabout way."

Not long ago, Kim Schmit's co-workers at a St. Cloud medical clinic bought a stone slab that features laser etchings of pictures of Greg and Josh hoisting beers. The photos were taken when the family visited Josh in Germany for his wedding.

The slab sits prominently inside Kim Schmit's home. The inscription reads: "You are now free and our tears wish you luck."

### In Unit Stalked by Suicide, Veterans Try to Save One Another

Members of a Marine battalion that served in a restive region in Afghanistan have been devastated by the deaths of comrades and frustrated by the V.A.

**By DAVE PHILIPPS - SEPT. 19, 2015**

After the sixth suicide in his old battalion, Manny Bojorquez sank onto his bed. With a half-empty bottle of Jim Beam beside him and a pistol in his hand, he began to cry.

He had gone to Afghanistan at 19 as a machine-gunner in the Marine Corps. In the 18 months since leaving the military, he had grown long hair and a bushy mustache. It was 2012. He was working part time in a store selling baseball caps and going to community college while living with his parents in the suburbs of Phoenix. He rarely mentioned the war to friends and family, and he never mentioned his nightmares.

He thought he was getting used to suicides in his old infantry unit, but the latest one had hit him like a brick: Joshua Markel, a mentor from his fire team, who had seemed unshakable. In Afghanistan, Corporal Markel volunteered for extra patrols and joked during firefights. Back home Mr. Markel appeared solid: a job with a sheriff's office, a new truck, a wife and time to hunt deer with his father. But that week, while watching football on TV with friends, he had wordlessly gone into his room, picked up a pistol and killed himself. He was 25.

Still reeling from the news, Mr. Bojorquez surveyed the old baseball posters on the walls of his childhood bedroom and the sun-bleached body armor hanging on his bedpost. Then he took a long pull from the bottle.

"If he couldn't make it," he recalled thinking to himself, "what chance do I have?"

He pressed the loaded pistol to his brow and pulled the trigger.

Mr. Bojorquez, 27, served in one of the hardest hit military units in Afghanistan, the Second Battalion, Seventh Marine Regiment. In 2008, the 2/7 deployed to a wild swath of Helmand Province. Well beyond reliable supply lines, the battalion regularly ran low on water and ammunition while coming under fire almost daily. During eight months of combat, the unit killed hundreds of enemy fighters and suffered more casualties than any other Marine battalion that year.

When its members returned, most left the military and melted back into the civilian landscape. They had families and played softball, taught high school and attended Ivy League universities. But many also struggled, unable to find solace. And for some, the agonies of war never ended.

Almost seven years after the deployment, suicide is spreading through the old unit like a virus. Of about 1,200 Marines who deployed with the 2/7 in 2008, at least 13 have killed themselves, two while on active duty, the rest after they left the military. The resulting suicide rate for the group is nearly four times the rate for young male veterans as a whole and 14 times that for all Americans.

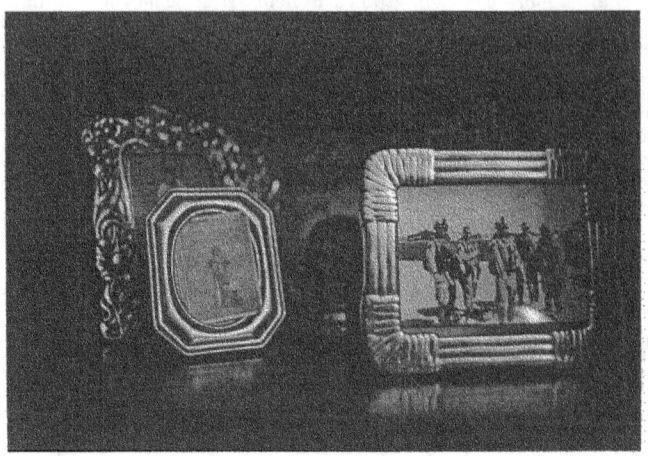

Photos of Manny Bojorquez, which his mother keeps at home, as a child and with members of the Second Battalion, Seventh Marine Regiment in Afghanistan. CreditTodd Heisler/The New York Times

The deaths started a few months after the Marines returned from the war in Afghanistan. A corporal put on his dress uniform and shot himself in his driveway. A former sergeant shot himself in front of his girlfriend and mother. An ex-sniper who pushed others to seek help for post-traumatic stress disorder shot himself while alone in his apartment.

The problem has grown over time. More men from the battalion killed themselves in 2014 - four - than in any previous year. Veterans of the unit, tightly connected by social media, sometimes learn of the deaths nearly as soon as they happen. In November, a 2/7 veteran of three combat tours posted a photo of his pistol on Snapchat with a note saying, "I miss you all." Minutes later, he killed himself.

The most recent suicide was in May, when Eduardo Bojorquez, no relation to Manny, overdosed on pills in his car. Men from the battalion converged from all over the country for his funeral in Las Vegas, filing silently past the grave, tossing roses that thumped on the plain metal coffin like drum beats.

"When the suicides started, I felt angry," Matt Havniear, a onetime lance corporal who carried a rocket launcher in the war, said in a phone interview from Oregon. "The next few, I would just be confused and sad. Then at about the 10th, I started feeling as if it was inevitable - that it is going to get us all and there is nothing we could do to stop it."

For years leaders at the top levels of the government have acknowledged the high suicide rate among veterans and spent heavily to try to reduce it. But the suicides have continued, and basic questions about who is most at risk and how best to help them are still largely unanswered. The authorities are not even aware of the spike in suicides in the 2/7; suicide experts at the Department of Veterans Affairs said they did not track suicide trends among veterans of specific military units. And the Marine Corps does not track suicides of former service members.

Feeling abandoned, members of the battalion have turned to a survival strategy they learned at war: depending on one another. Doing what the government has not, they have used free software and social media to create a quick-response system that allows them to track, monitor and intervene with some of their most troubled comrades.

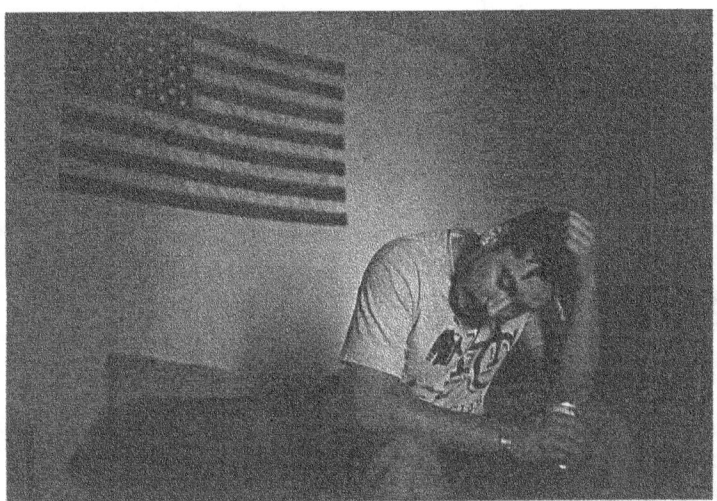

Manny Bojorquez, 27, in the living room of his apartment in Mesa, Ariz. CreditTodd Heisler/The New York Times

Their system has made a few saves, but many in the battalion still feel stalked by suicide.

"To this day I'm scared of it," said Ruben Sevilla, 28, who deployed twice with the 2/7 and now works for a warehouse management company called Legacy SCS near Chicago. "If all these guys can do that, what's stopping me? That's what freaks me out the most. I haven't touched a gun since I got out of the Marine Corps because I'm afraid to."

The morning after Manny Bojorquez tried to shoot himself in 2012, he opened his eyes to sunlight streaming in his window and found the loaded gun on the floor. Through his whiskey headache, he pieced together that his gun had jammed and that he had passed out drunk.

A week later, he stood alongside more than a dozen other Marine veterans at Mr. Markel's funeral in Lincoln, Neb. The crack of rifles echoed off the headstones as an honor guard fired a salute.

Mr. Bojorquez offered his condolences to Mr. Markel's mother after the funeral. He thought about how life seemed increasingly bitter. The thrill of combat was gone. Only regrets and flashbacks remained.

Mr. Markel's mother pressed something into Mr. Bojorquez's palm at the funeral, a spent brass shell casing from the honor guard. Promise me, she said to him, that you will never put your mother through this. Mr. Bojorquez promised.

That began a three-year odyssey in which the deaths of his friends weighed on Mr. Bojorquez, who tried repeatedly to get help from Veterans Affairs but ultimately gave up.

"I was lost then. I still am kind of lost," he said in a recent interview. "I was just trying to look for something that wasn't there. I was trying to look for an answer that I don't have - that no one does."

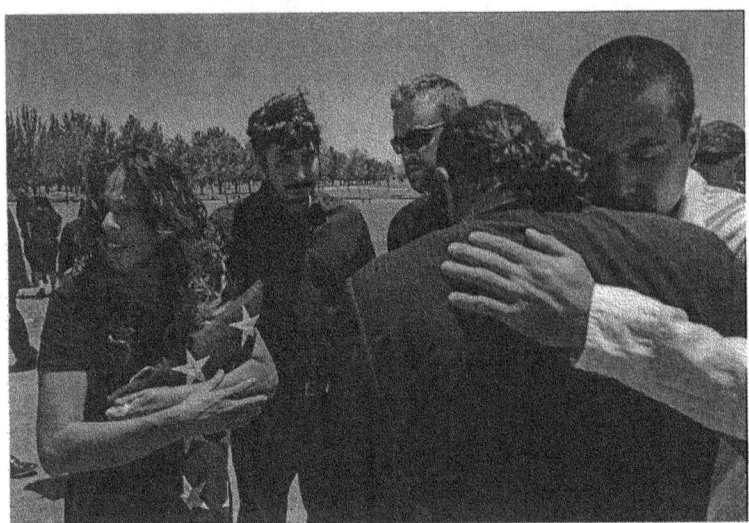

Manny Bojorquez, second from left, at the funeral of Eduardo Bojorquez, a member of the 2/7 who took his own life in May. The two men were not related.CreditTodd Heisler/The New York Times

He was wearing a bracelet etched with the names of four Marines: one who died on the battlefield and three who died by their own hands at home.

*'The Forgotten Battalion'*

In Afghanistan, after the men of the 2/7 realized the scope of their mission, they began calling themselves "the Forgotten Battalion."

In the spring of 2008, they deployed from their base at Twenty-Nine Palms, Calif., to an untamed stretch of Afghanistan surrounding the city of Sangin.

Their job was to pacify a Taliban stronghold the size of Massachusetts that had never been controlled by coalition troops, or anyone else. Opium poppies grew in fields as vast as those of corn in the Midwest. Roads were pocked with the rusting hulks of Soviet tanks destroyed in a different war.

The Marines were spread out in sandbag outposts, hours from reinforcements, and often outnumbered. With the Pentagon focused on the surge in Iraq, equipment was scant. There was no dedicated air support, few mine-sweeping trucks, often no refrigeration. The only reliable abundance was combat.

"Machine guns, mortars, rockets, RPGs, I.E.D.s, constant fighting. It was like the Wild West," said Keith Branch of Austin, Tex., who was a 20-year-old rifleman who patrolled a village called Now Zad.

In that village alone, two Marine platoons fired more than 2,500 mortar rounds, called in 50,000 pounds of explosives from aircraft and killed 185 enemy fighters, battalion documents show.

Many of the Marines had deployed to Iraq just eight months before. At least two had been shot by snipers and one was hit by a grenade in Iraq, but they were redeployed to Afghanistan anyway. All three later killed themselves.

The I.E.D.s, or improvised explosive devices, plagued patrols. The first convoy arriving in Sangin hit two. In the next two weeks, an I.E.D. hidden in a bicycle killed a medic, an I.E.D. packed in a culvert killed three Marines in a Humvee, and an I.E.D. discovered in a dirt lane killed a specialist trained to defuse the explosives.

Manny Bojorquez spent the tour in a village called Musa Qala, where repeated offensives failed to drive out the Taliban.

One evening his squad was patrolling single file across a field when the enemy ambushed it on two sides. As the squad sprinted for cover, Mr. Bojorquez watched a bullet hit a Marine in front of him, who crumpled to the dirt. Mr. Bojorquez and another Marine grabbed the bleeding man and dragged him to a ditch.

Pressed against the ground, readying his machine gun, Mr. Bojorquez looked over and saw his teammate Corporal Markel laying down fire - with a steady grin on his face. Together they showered the surrounding fields and houses with bullets, providing cover for a medic. But the enemy pressed harder, another Marine was hit and the outnumbered squad had to pick up and run.

"It's funny. I was never scared. You just act. But it stuck with me," Mr. Bojorquez said.

By the end of the deployment, 20 Marines in the battalion had been killed and 140 had been wounded. Many lost limbs. Some were badly burned; others were so battered by blasts that they can scarcely function day to day.

Others returned unscathed, but unable to fall in with civilian life. Members of the battalion say what they brought home from combat is more complex than just PTSD. Many regret things they did - or failed to do. Some feel betrayed that the deep sacrifices made in combat seem to have achieved little. Others cannot reconcile the stark intensity of war with home's mannered expectations, leaving them alienated among family and friends. It is not just symptoms like sleeplessness or flashbacks, but an injury to their sense of self.

**Where to Call for Help**

The Department of Veterans Affairs maintains a hotline for veterans in crisis that operates 24 hours a day. Call 1–800–273–8255 and press 1. Online, visit veteranscrisisline.net/chat, or send a text message to 838255.

"Something happens over there," said Mr. Havniear, whose best friend from the battalion tried suicide by cutting his wrists after returning home, but survived. "You wake up a primal part of your brain you are not supposed to listen to, and it becomes a part of you. I shot an old woman. I shot her on purpose because she was running at us with an RPG. You see someone blown in half, or you carry a foot. You can try, but it is hard to get away from that."

After Mr. Bojorquez returned home, he started having a recurring nightmare. He was patrolling with his squad when bomb blasts killed everyone but him. As the dust cleared, he looked up to see enemy fighters surging forward. He often sat up in bed, thinking he was choking on his own blood.

*One Mission's Toll*

Beginning in 2005, suicide rates among Iraq and Afghanistan veterans started to climb sharply, and the military and Veterans Affairs created a number of programs to fight the problem. Despite spending hundreds of millions on research, the department and the military still know little about how combat experience affects suicide risk, according to suicide researchers focused on the military.

Many recent studies have focused on whether deployment was a risk factor for suicide, and found that it was not.

The results appeared to show something paradoxical: Those deployed to war were actually less likely to commit suicide. But critics of the studies say most people deployed in war zones do not face enemy fire. The risk for true combat veterans is hidden in the larger results, and has never been properly examined, they assert.

"They may have 10 times the risk, they may have 100 times, and we don't know, because no one has looked," said Michael Schoenbaum, an epidemiologist at the Centers for Disease Control and Prevention.

The men of the 2/7 overwhelmingly see a tie between combat and their suicide problem. Not only were all of the men who committed suicide young infantrymen who struggled with experiences of killing and loss, they say, but it is possible to trace one traumatic moment forward and see how those involved are now struggling.

Noel Guerrero and Manny Bojorquez were best friends in the battalion. As two Mexican-Americans from the Southwest, they bonded in infantry school over a love of Mexican hot sauce. In Afghanistan, they would share bottles sent from home.

On one mission, Mr. Guerrero, then a 20-year-old lance corporal, was a machine-gunner atop a truck at the lead of a supply convoy. He said he was good at finding I.E.D.s and over six months had spotted almost a dozen that the battalion was able to avoid. But one day, the truck hit a big one, and the explosion flung him against his gun turret.

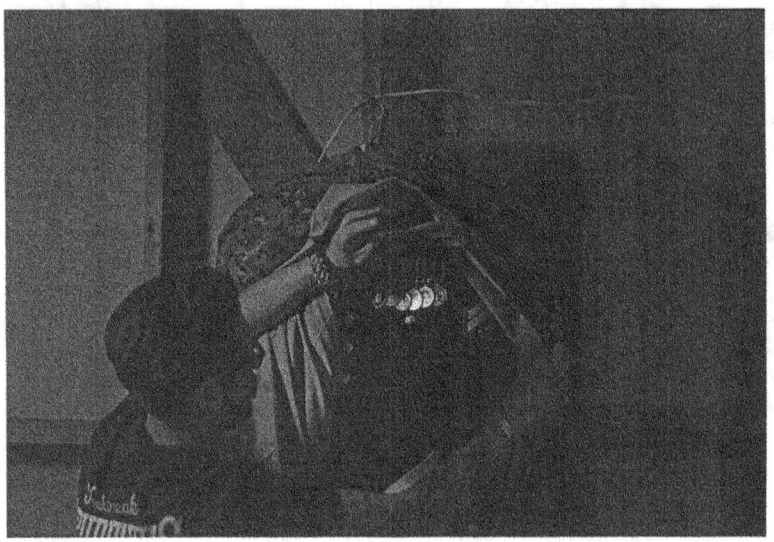

Noel Guerrero keeps his dress uniform, with his Purple Heart, in his garage. Mr. Guerrero, 28, said the war had left him with "a dark shadow you can never take away."CreditTodd Heisler/The New York Times

Mr. Guerrero crawled from the smoking vehicle, his head spinning. He watched his sergeant's Humvee roll in to help. Then suddenly, another blast swallowed the sergeant's truck in smoke. The truck shot up 10 feet and came down with a crash, falling to its side. Then, chaos. The driver was trapped and screaming, with his arm caught under the wreckage. A medic in the back was pinned by a seat crushed against the truck's ceiling. The sergeant was dead.

Before Mr. Guerrero could get to his feet to help, enemy fire started thudding into the ground around him. He spotted his machine gun in the dirt, where it had landed after being blown out of the truck, and with his vision still blurred, he began to return fire.

Two other Marines, Cpl. Jastin Pak and Lance Cpl. Tanner Cleveland, scrambled into the wreckage. Mr. Pak crouched over the driver, shielding him until a line of Marines could lift the truck enough to free his arm. Mr. Pak and Mr. Cleveland emerged covered with blood, clutching the wounded, then went back for the remains of the sergeant. The platoon was out of body bags, so they stuffed the sergeant's remains into a sleeping bag.

When it was all over, Mr. Guerrero picked up a cigarette that had been blown out of one of the trucks and lit it. After he exhaled, he noticed it was spotted with blood. He smoked it anyway.

Since that day, Mr. Guerrero has blamed himself for the ordeal and has tried to kill himself three times. Mr. Cleveland, 26, of Chicago, also tried suicide, and Mr. Pak, of Oceanside, Calif., hanged himself in November.

"You come back and try to be a normal kid, but there is always a shadow on you, a dark shadow you can never take away," Mr. Guerrero, now 28, said in an interview at his home in San Diego.

"Now, when I meet someone, I already know what they look like dead. I can't help but think that way. And I ask myself, 'Do I want to live with this feeling for the rest of my life, or is it better to just finish it off?' "

*Lacking Data on Suicides*

The first few suicides struck the men of the battalion as random. It was only over time that they came to see the deaths as a part of their war story - combat deaths that happened after the fact.

Cpl. Richard McShan died first. He had survived a truck bomb in Iraq before deploying to Afghanistan. Four months after they returned, in the spring of 2009, he put on his dress uniform after an argument with his girlfriend and shot himself in his driveway.

In December 2009, Pfc. Christopher G. Stewart hanged himself from a door in his barracks.

In April 2010, Shawn Jensen, a sergeant who had just gotten out of the Marines and moved home to rural Washington State to work in construction, shot himself during an argument with his girlfriend and mother.

The Marines tended to chalk up these first suicides to foolish impulses or prewar problems. Then came the death that shook the battalion, and prompted many to ask whether something was wrong not just with the men who killed themselves, but with them all.

## Battalion Suicides

Thirteen Marines who deployed with the Second Battalion, Seventh Marine Regiment to Afghanistan in 2008 later killed themselves. All were young, low-ranking infantry troops.

**APRIL 1, 2009**
Cpl. Richard McShan, 23

**DEC. 23, 2009**
Pvt. Christopher G. Stewart, 21

**APRIL 3, 2010**
Sgt. Shawn Jensen, 27

**MARCH 31, 2011**
Cpl. Clay Hunt, 28

**JULY 1, 2012**
Cpl. Jeremie Ross, 25

**OCT. 6, 2012**
Cpl. Joshua Markel, 25

**DEC. 9, 2012**
Lance Cpl. Ufrano Rios Jimenez, 23

**JAN. 18, 2013**
Cpl. Luis Rocha, 23

**APRIL 12, 2014**
Cpl. Elias Reyes Jr., 27

**OCT. 6, 2014**
Lance Cpl. Tyler Wilkerson, 27

**NOV. 2, 2014**
Cpl. Joseph Gellings, 29

**NOV. 5, 2014**
Sgt. Jastin Pak, 27

**MAY 30, 2015**
Lance Cpl. Eduardo Bojorquez, 25

Cpl. Clay Hunt had been a sniper in the battalion. After he got out of the Marine Corps in 2009 after his second tour, his disenchantment with the war grew, and he sought treatment from Veterans Affairs for depression and PTSD.

He became an outspoken advocate for young veterans, speaking openly about his problems and lobbying for better care for veterans on Capitol Hill. In 2010, he was featured in a public service message urging veterans to seek support from their comrades.

At the same time, Mr. Hunt was fighting to get adequate care at the V.A., encountering long delays and inconsistent treatment, according to his mother, Susan Selke of Houston.

Friends said Mr. Hunt had felt directionless. "There is so much isolation and lack of purpose. We came home from war unprepared for peace, and we've had to find a new mission," said Jake Wood, who was also a sniper in the 2/7. "He struggled to do that."

Mr. Hunt shot himself in his apartment in Texas in March 2011. He was 28.

After years of lobbying by his family and veterans' groups, Congress in February passed the Clay Hunt Suicide Prevention for American Veterans Act, which provides additional suicide prevention resources for Veterans Affairs.

"When he died, all the guys, we couldn't understand it," said Danny Kwan of San Gabriel, Calif., an ex-corporal who served two tours with Mr. Hunt. "He had done exactly what he had been fighting against."

At the time of Mr. Hunt's suicide, Mr. Kwan was fresh out of the Marines. One night when he was drunk and despondent over a recent breakup, he put a gun to his head and pulled the trigger. He jerked the gun away as it fired, sending the bullet through a wall.

"At the last moment I decided I wanted to live," Mr. Kwan said. "We all have our demons. Some more than others."

No one knows whether the battalion's suicide rate is abnormally high or a common trait of fighting units hit hard by combat, because no one monitors troops over time. In an era of Big Data, when algorithms can predict human patterns in startling detail, suicide data for veterans is incomplete and years old by the time it is available. The most recentdata is from 2011.

The Department of Veterans Affairs and the Pentagon say they have introduced a new system, called the Suicide Data Repository, that is faster and more complete.

But Dr. Harold Kudler, chief mental health consultant to the department, said the military and V.A. did not share information that could allow the monitoring of combat units over time.

"Might that be a good idea? It might be a good idea," he said. "But it's not in our ability to achieve. It's not our mission."

*A Pact to Help*

In December 2012, Marines from the 2/7 converged on a small town in the Central Valley of California for another funeral. A former radioman named Ufrano Rios Jimenez had killed himself with a shot to the heart.

Mr. Rios had lost a leg in Afghanistan. Once home, he struggled with PTSD. But he gave up on treatment at the V.A. and turned to alcohol, painkillers and eventually heroin, according to his former girlfriend, Allison Keefer. After the suicide of a friend from the battalion, Jeremie Ross, in July 2012, he quit work and slipped into a deep depression.

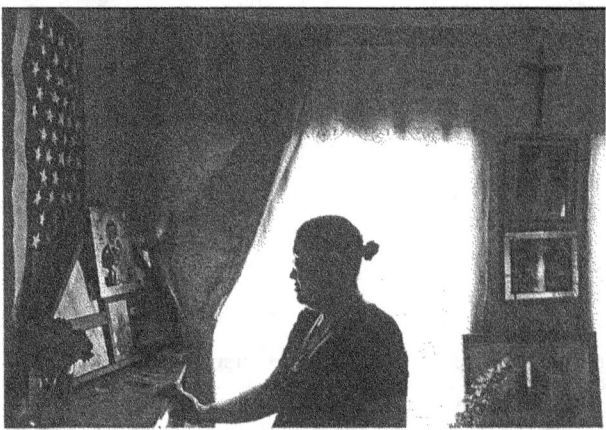

Maria T. Jauregui stood by the shrine to her son, Elias Reyes Jr., that she keeps at her home in Los Angeles. CreditTodd Heisler/The New York Times

At the funeral, Mr. Bojorquez stood with the others from the 2/7 as they shook their heads and discussed what to do. A battle-hardened former corporal named Travis Wilkerson spoke up.

Once a fearsome team leader in a deadly sector of Sangin, he was now working as a night manager at a sandwich shop. He was one of several men from the battalion who had changed their lives radically in search of peace, growing a bushy beard and taking a vow of nonviolence.

"Real talk, guys, let's make a pact, right here," Travis Wilkerson said. "I don't want to go to any more funerals. Let's promise to reach out and talk. Get your phones out, put my number in. Call me day or night. I'm not doing this again."

His twin brother, Tyler Wilkerson, who had served in the same platoon, stood next to him. After the Marines, he had become a Buddhist and joined Greenpeace. He said he agreed.

Then a three-tour former corporal named Elias Reyes Jr. stepped forward. He had a long ponytail and a degree in philosophy from the University of California, Los Angeles. He was hoping to attend medical school.

Enough of this, he said. One by one, the others joined the pact.

Just over a year later, Mr. Reyes killed himself. In combat, he had been flattened by explosions several times and seen friends maimed and killed.

Back home, he was getting counseling at the V.A., family members said, but faced delays and struggled to find a therapist who he felt understood him. In April 2014, he hanged himself in his apartment.

"He was very religious, a Catholic," his sister, Margarita Reyes, said. "To do what he did, he must have been in so much pain."

News of his death was one more in a mounting pile of problems for Tyler Wilkerson.

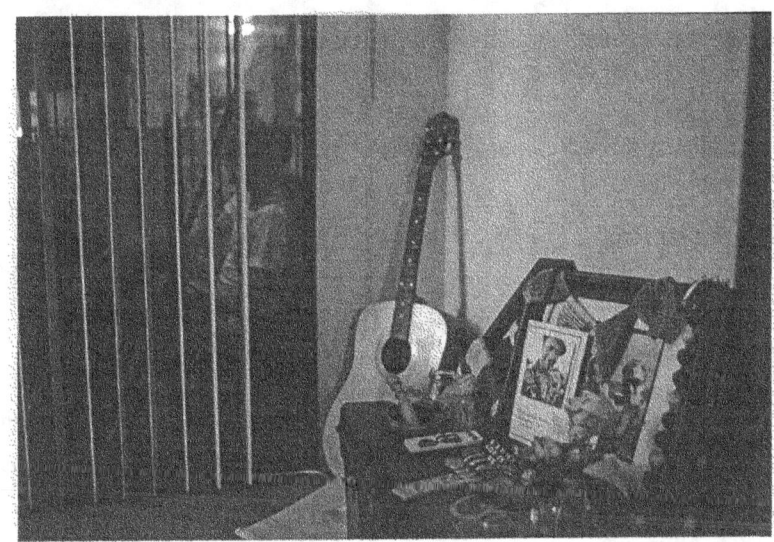

A shrine to Tyler Wilkerson, kept by his twin brother, Travis, left, sitting on a balcony at his home in San Diego. CreditTodd Heisler/The New York Times

After the Marines, Tyler Wilkerson, also a Californian, became part of a commandolike team of Greenpeace protesters. The job combined his love of tactical missions and his vow of nonviolence.

But in March 2013, he was arrested after he and others trespassed to unfurl giant banners that accused Procter & Gamble, the household products company, of destroying rain forests.

In the months that followed, his girlfriend broke up with him and Greenpeace fired him, leaving him alone with wartime memories that he had tried to escape.

He fatally shot himself in October 2014, a few weeks before he was to stand trial for the Greenpeace action.

"He felt like he had lost everything," Travis Wilkerson said. "He said his life looked like this endless mountain he couldn't see the top of."

Other deaths soon followed.

A month later, a mortar man who had served three tours at war, Joseph Gellings, killed himself at his home in Kansas.

He had tried mental health treatment at the V.A., but gave up after delays and other frustrations, according to his longtime girlfriend, Jenna Passio. Instead, she said, he drank and became reclusive. She eventually left him, taking their daughter.

After their breakup, he posted to Facebook, "I'm done with life." Other Marines texted and called to check on him.

"Disregard guys, everything is fine," he replied.

A short time later he shot himself in the head as Ms. Passio looked on in horror. Realizing he was only wounded, he went into a bathroom in his home and shot himself again.

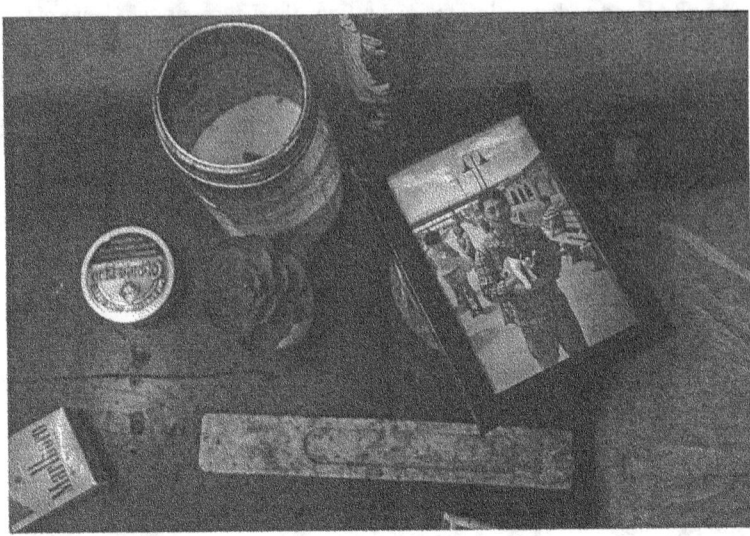

A shrine dedicated to Jastin Pak at the home of Dimitri Karras, who was a Marine comrade, in Oceanside, Calif. CreditTodd Heisler/The New York Times

As the news rocketed across Facebook the next day, Mr. Cleveland, who had tried suicide, thought, "It's to the point now where it's like, 'Who is next?' "

It was the friend who had helped Mr. Cleveland pull body parts from a smoldering Humvee in Afghanistan, Jastin Pak. Three days after Mr. Gellings's death, Mr. Pak, 27, hanged himself from a pine tree in the mountains west of his home.

On his desk, Mr. Pak left a completed "stressful incident form" that the veterans hospital in San Diego gave him on his initial visit a few days before. It asked him to list events from combat that were causing him anguish. He filled two pages, starting with the killing of an older man in Iraq who had been unarmed and finishing with placing the remains of the dead sergeant into a sleeping bag.

*Failed Therapy*

After the eighth suicide in the battalion, in 2013, Mr. Bojorquez decided he needed professional help and made an appointment at the veterans hospital in Phoenix.

He sat down with a therapist, a young woman. After listening for a few minutes, she told him that she knew he was hurting, but that he would just have to get over the deaths of his friends. He should treat it, he recalled her saying, "like a bad breakup with a girl."

The comment caught him like a hook. Guys he knew had been blown to pieces and burned to death. One came home with shrapnel in his face from a friend's skull. Now they were killing themselves at an alarming rate. And the therapist wanted him to get over it like a breakup?

Mr. Bojorquez shot out of his seat and began yelling. "What are you talking about?" he said. "This isn't something you just get over."

He had tried getting help at the V.A. once before, right after Mr. Markel's funeral, and had walked out when he realized the counselor had not read his file. Now he was angry that he had returned. With each visit, it appeared to him that the professionals trained to make sense of what he was feeling understood it less than he did.

He threw a chair across the room and stomped out, vowing again never to go back to the V.A.

In recent years, suicide prevention efforts by the Department of Veterans Affairs have focused on encouraging veterans to go to its hospitals for help, but a bigger problem could be keeping them there.

In interviews, many Marines from the battalion said they received effective care at the V.A. But many others said they had quit the treatment because of what they considered long waits, ineffective therapists and doctors' overreliance on drugs.

Six of the 13 Marines from the battalion who committed suicide had tried and then given up on V.A. treatment, discouraged by the bureaucracy and poor results, according to friends and relatives.

A 2014 study of 204,000 veterans, in The Journal of the American Psychiatric Association, found nearly two-thirds of Iraq and Afghanistan veterans stopped Veterans Affairs therapy for PTSD within a year, before completing the treatment. A smaller study from the same year found about 90 percent dropped out of therapy.

The therapies, considered by the department to be the gold standard of evidence-based treatments, rely on having patients repeatedly revisit traumatic memories - remembrances that seem to cause many to quit. Evaluations of the effectiveness of the programs often do not account for the large number of patients who find the process disturbing and drop out.

Dr. Kudler of the Department of Veterans Affairs said data showed that 28 percent of patients drop out of PTSD therapy, but that most veterans stay in treatment and report improvements.

He added that dropout is an issue in all mental health care, not just among veterans, and that the department was constantly trying to provide alternative types of therapy, like meditation.

Craig J. Bryan, a psychologist and an Iraq war veteran, said that "the V.A. has done more to try to prevent suicide than anyone has done in the history of the human race." Mr. Bryan, who runs the National Center for Veterans Studies at the University of Utah, added: "But most veterans who kill themselves do not go to treatment or give up. They are not interested. That is the challenge."

Mr. Bojorquez tried the system one more time out of desperation. After the spate of suicides in 2014, he called and said he needed help. The V.A. had him see a psychologist and psychiatrist.

He told them that he wanted therapy but no drugs. Too many friends had stories of bad reactions. One, Luis Rocha, had taken a photograph of all his pill bottles right before shooting himself.

"We get it, no drugs," he recalled them saying. But on his way out, after scheduling a return appointment in two months, he was handed a bag filled with bottles of pills. He calmly walked to his car, then screamed and pounded the steering wheel.

He wanted to get better, so he started taking the medications - an antidepressant, an anti-anxiety drug and a drug to help him sleep - but they made him feel worse, he said. His nightmares grew more vivid, his urge to kill himself more urgent.

After a few weeks, he flushed the pills down the toilet, determined to deal with his problems on his own.

*Fighting the Label*

Increasingly, members of the battalion felt that at home, as in Afghanistan, they were still the Forgotten Battalion. So they looked for help from the people they counted on in Afghanistan: their fellow Marines.

In November, Mr. Branch, who was completing a degree in social work in Texas, posted a request on Facebook asking the others to enter their addresses in a Google spreadsheet. That way, if a Marine in Montana was worried about a friend in Georgia, he could look on the spreadsheet and find someone nearby to help.

"All of us are going through the same struggle," Mr. Branch, now 28, said in an interview. "If we can get someone there that a guy can relate to, we hope it will make all the difference."

The spreadsheet is part of a wider realization among young veterans that connecting with other veterans - whether through volunteering, sports, art or other shared experiences - can be potent medicine.

One battalion member started an organic farm intended to help veterans heal by growing food. Another leads trips to bring together veterans with PTSD. Mr. Wood, 32, the former sniper, founded a national network of veterans, called Team Rubicon, that provides volunteer relief work after natural disasters.

"We did it because we really wanted to help others," said Mr. Wood, of Los Angeles. "We soon realized it would help us, too."

Less than two weeks after the Google spreadsheet was created, a text message popped up on the phone of a Marine veteran named Geoff Kamp. It was just after 11 p.m. on a Wednesday in November.

Mr. Kamp, who had turned in early to be up for his shift with the Postal Service, reached for the phone next to his bed, read the text, turned to his wife and said, "I'm going to be gone for a while."

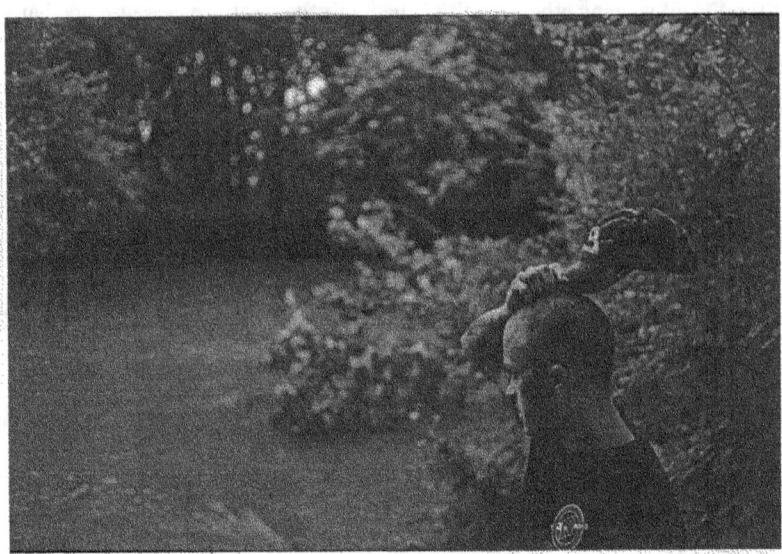

Charles Gerard, a member of 2/7, by Wildcat Creek, a place he likes to visit near his home in Rossville, Ind.CreditTodd Heisler/The New York Times

An hour earlier, a 27-year-old Marine veteran, Charles Gerard, had changed his Facebook profile photo to an image of a rifle stuck in the dirt, topped with a helmet - the symbol of someone killed in action. In a post, he wrote: "I can't do it anymore."

After surviving an ambush in Afghanistan where several Marines were injured, Mr. Gerard said, he was treated for PTSD by the Marine Corps. But when his enlistment ended in 2011, so did his therapy. He tried to continue at the V.A., but long delays meant it was two years before he got any treatment, and even then, he said, he found it ineffective.

He moved back to rural Indiana and worked at factories, but his anger frayed ties with his friends and family. News that comrades from the battalion had killed themselves pushed him deeper into despair. The night he changed his profile picture, his girlfriend had left him.

Within minutes, the battalion's response system kicked in. Mr. Havniear in Oregon spotted the Facebook post and called a Marine in Utah who had been Mr. Gerard's roommate. They called Mr. Gerard immediately but got no answer. Mr. Gerard was parked in his pickup by a lake outside of town with a hunting rifle in his lap.

Desperate to head off another death, they opened the Google spreadsheet and found Mr. Kamp, 90 minutes away. Within 10 minutes, he was in his truck, speeding north through the late autumn corn stubble.

Mr. Kamp had never met Mr. Gerard. But he, too, had been injured in a firefight, and been dogged by guilt and anger afterward.

"Every one of the guys that's died, I see myself in them," he said later in an interview at his home. "It's like you are always just one bad day away from that being you."

At the lake, Mr. Gerard propped his rifle against his head, closed his eyes and pulled the trigger. There was a click, then nothing.

He took a deep breath and checked the chamber. It was loaded, but the round was a dud.

He decided the universe was telling him it was not his time to die. He tossed his remaining ammunition in the lake and drove home.

A few minutes later, Mr. Kamp knocked on the door.

They talked on the couch most of the night about relationships, work, mortgages, combat, guys who did not make it home and the cold feeling after Afghanistan that you are alone even when surrounded by other people.

"We'll make it through this," Mr. Kamp told him.

Mr. Kamp eventually called the sheriff's office for help, took the rifle for safe-keeping and stayed until paramedics took Mr. Gerard to the veterans hospital in Indianapolis.

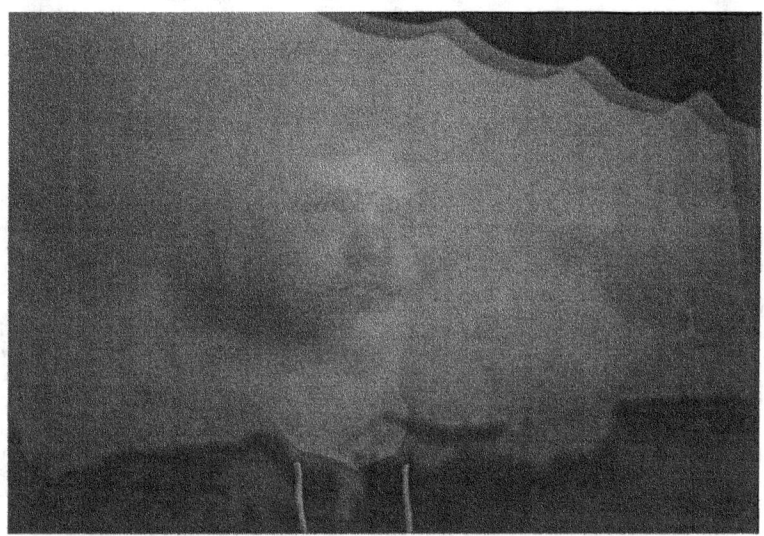

Geoff Kamp went to Mr. Gerard's aid after being notified by the 2/7's alert system on social media.CreditTodd Heisler/The New York Times

In March, members of the group used their informal network to intervene with another battalion member in Louisiana. The jury-rigged system is far from ideal, they said, but they are determined to make it work.

Mr. Gerard's experience shows, however, that the system is only as good as the V.A. treatment it is intended to connect to. The night he went to the psychiatric ward at the Indianapolis veterans hospital, he said, he waited and waited for a doctor to see him. After 24 hours, he gave up and checked himself out.

"There was no one there for me," Mr. Gerard said in a quiet voice during a recent interview at his home after a 12-hour night shift at an auto plant.

He looked pale and gaunt, a far cry from the tan and muscular Marine in photos from Afghanistan. Garbage and unwashed dishes were piled up around him. The curtains were drawn.

He crushed out a cigarette. The V.A.? "I've had nothing to do with them since," he said.

*A Lifesaving Call*

After swearing off the V.A., Manny Bojorquez turned increasingly to friends for support. Late-night calls and texts with guys from the battalion seemed to help more than therapy ever did.

He reconnected with Mr. Guerrero, who still shared his love of Mexican hot sauce. The machine-gunner was living in California, in his last year of college, and he had a baby boy.

"The guys we served with, they are the only ones we can really talk to," Mr. Bojorquez said in an interview.

But in November, Mr. Bojorquez got a text from Mr. Guerrero that upended everything. "I don't think I can do this life anymore," it said.

Mr. Guerrero had never mentioned it to others, but he still believed his sergeant's death was his fault. If only he had yelled a warning. Or spotted the I.E.D. He was getting therapy and medication for his depression, but still often woke up with a deep dread, as if he were sitting at the principal's office, waiting to be punished. Every day, he wore a bracelet etched with the sergeant's name.

64

That night, Mr. Guerrero had been watching television with his wife after church when something snapped. He crumpled to the floor and backed into a corner, crying, "I'm sorry, I'm sorry."

He had not smoked since the Marines, but pleaded with his wife to go out and buy cigarettes. The panic and guilt were so excruciating that he decided the only relief was to kill himself. He went onto his porch with shaking hands to text Mr. Bojorquez to say goodbye.

Mr. Bojorquez called immediately. Mr. Guerrero picked up, sobbing, but after a few words hung up.

A fear had crept over Mr. Bojorquez over the last year that he was doomed to watch his friends die one after another until he was the only one left. At times, he saw it as another reason to kill himself. But it was also motivation to break the pattern.

He knew he had to call 911, but hesitated. The call might land Mr. Guerrero in a psychiatric ward or ruin his marriage, already strained. Worse, if the police barged in, his friend might go berserk. Someone could get hurt. But what choice was there?

The police pounded on the door just as Mr. Guerrero put a handful of pills into his mouth. He spent the next few weeks in a private inpatient treatment program for PTSD.

It was far from a cure. He said he was still deeply depressed and ashamed. He still slept on the couch instead of in his wife's bed, and he was not speaking to his parents. But he was alive.

Six weeks later, Mr. Bojorquez drove out to visit him in San Diego. The 911 call had not broken their friendship, but it had broken the long silence in which neither mentioned what he had brought home from war.

They greeted each other in a hug. During a lunch at a nearby taqueria, Mr. Bojorquez talked about the night he had put a gun to his head. Mr. Guerrero talked about watching his sergeant's Humvee explode and being so rattled afterward that he did not care that his cigarette was flecked with blood. They stayed long after the lunch crowd cleared out.

"This is good - us here like this," Mr. Guerrero told his friend. "It's the times when I'm alone that I fear."

They had found small ways to rebuild their lives. Mr. Guerrero had become a rabid marathoner and was leading the youth band at his church. Mr. Bojorquez was studying to join the United States Border Patrol and playing on a softball team with his brother.

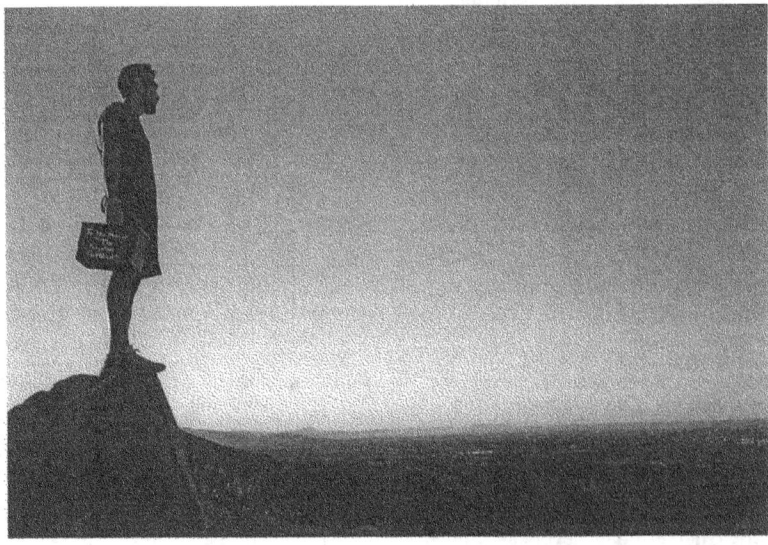

Mr. Guerrero on a mountain in San Diego at dawn, holding an ammunition box that he keeps there for Marines who want to leave letters or sign their names.CreditTodd Heisler/The New York Times

At dawn the next morning, Mr. Guerrero took Mr. Bojorquez on his favorite run to the top of a mountain behind his house. He had placed an old metal ammunition box at the top, where Marines could leave letters and sign their names. He dedicated it to the men of the Forgotten Battalion.

As they clambered up the trail, they talked about how hard it was to find balance.

"The death of my brothers consumes me," Mr. Guerrero said between breaths. "It gives me this dark energy. I don't know what to do, so I run. I run all the time. I pray I never run out of trails to run."

It was five winding miles to the summit. When they reached it, the two stood side by side catching their breath and looking out at the dawn spreading over the ocean. Mr. Bojorquez hung his arm over his friend's shoulder. Hummingbirds zipped through the pink light.

Mr. Guerrero broke the silence.

"I'm glad I got to share this with you," he told his friend. "I wish I could bring the whole battalion up here."

### Correction: September 23, 2015

An article on Sunday about the high number of suicides among a Marine battalion that served in Afghanistan misidentified the association that sponsored a 2014 study of 204,000 veterans on post-traumatic stress disorder. It is the American Psychiatric Association, not the American Psychological Association.

The Department of Veterans Affairs maintains a hotline for veterans in crisis that operates 24 hours a day. Call 1–800–273–8255 and press 1, go to veteranscrisisline.net/chat, or send a text to 838255.

A version of this article appears in print on September 20, 2015, on page A1 of the New York edition with the headline: A Unit Stalked by Suicide, Trying to Save Itself.

### Prepared Statement of Jacqueline Maffucci, Ph.D.

Chairman Miller, Ranking Member Brown and Distinguished Members of the Committee:

On behalf of Iraq and Afghanistan Veterans of America (IAVA) and our more than 425,000 members, thank you for the opportunity to share our views on the Department of Veterans' Affairs efforts to reduce suicide among veterans.

In 2014, IAVA launched the Campaign to Combat Suicide. This was a result of our members continually identifying mental health and suicide as the number one issue facing post-9/11 veterans in our annual membership survey. This campaign centers around the principle that timely access to high quality mental health care is critical in the fight to combat veteran suicides.

The signing of the Clay Hunt SAV Act into law was an important first step to addressing this. We thank you for your support of this legislation, the VA for their commitment to fully implement this law and Richard and Susan Selke for courageously uniting us all to do the right thing. We knew it would take time to do so correctly and we've been pleased that the VA's Mental Health Service team has included us in that process. While progress has seemingly been slow, we expected that this first year would be spent laying the foundation to implement the law and identifying funds to do so. We look forward to continuing to be a part of the implementation while working with the VA and Congress to continue working towards progress on this issue with new initiatives.

I'd like to focus today on four specific areas that IAVA feels are critical to this progress: Access to Care; Interdisciplinary Approach to Care; Research; and Supporting Those Most at Risk.

### Access to High Quality Mental Health Care

IAVA's Rapid Response Referral Program connects veterans and their family members to quality resources. Mental health and suicide challenges are among the top three issues our team is responding to.

In our most recent annual membership survey, over half of the respondents reported having a mental health injury and over 80 percent reported seeking care for that injury. For over 75 percent, the impact of a loved one suggesting they seek help made a huge difference and resulted in them finding that help. For IAVA this is a good news story. More of our members are seeking help, and the role of family and friends taking that first step is huge.

For those in care, three out of four are using the VA. And this year, we saw over 75 percent of those using VA mental health report little to no challenges scheduling an appointment, up 10 percent compared to last year and comparable with those using a non-VA clinician. The same number were also satisfied with that care.

The challenge associated with growing awareness of service-related mental health challenges and this improved care is an increase in demand for high quality mental health care rising both in- and outside of the VA. It is critical to ensure that the VA is properly resourced to provide high quality mental health care; a challenge made even more difficult by the dwindling supply of mental health professionals.

Efforts are underway to bolster the number of mental health professionals. The Secretary is carrying out the ever important task of recruiting medical students into the VA. Joining Forces has been critical in urging medical schools to improve curricula to ensure that that these students are better equipped to care for veterans and their families. But that's not enough.

Beyond the challenge of a clinician shortage is the difficult task of hiring and retaining talent in VA. A recent VA OIG report that looked at hiring and loss rates of VA psychologists found that a significant percentage of the total gains from hiring was offset by losses.[1] The VA needs to fully understand and address the reasons that staff leave and how to best attract and retain new talent. They need to do so with the knowledge of where the demand is for those professionals using updated models and real time data.

The federal hiring process can also be confusing and lengthy, which can deter candidates. And the VA itself, particularly in today's climate, can be a challenging place to work. We often forget to praise the talented and dedicated staff who sacrifice in service of the VA's mission, some of whom are IAVA members themselves. IAVA members have shared stories with me of the great work and dedication of these staff, telling me how these individuals have saved their lives or cared for them in some of their hardest moments. We all must do our part to help celebrate what makes the VA good while also focusing on how to make it better.

Finally, we need to ensure high quality care outside the VA as well. Just under 40 percent of the total veteran population seek care at the VA, which means the current community clinical workforce needs to be equipped to support veterans and their families. A recent RAND report estimates that only eight percent of community mental health providers are prepared to address the mental health needs of this population.[2] It is not even standard practice to ask if a patient is has served in the military. This has got to change. New Hampshire is leading the way with its campaign, "Ask the Question." But beyond asking the question, providers need to know how best to provide treatment once they have the answer. The VA and its partners (particularly its academic partners) are best equipped to lead this effort.

**Interdisciplinary Approach to Care**

But suicide prevention is not just about mental health care. In February, the VA hosted a Suicide Prevention Summit, and IAVA and Vietnam Veterans of America were both invited to speak. Together, we called upon the Secretary to elevate the VA's Suicide Prevention Office from Clinical Operations under Mental Health Services in VHA to the Office of the Secretary, at the same level that DOD places the office in its structure. Our reasoning is simple: while mental health is a major aspect of suicide prevention, it is not the only aspect. There are social factors that can also impact these actions, factors such as employment, finances and social supports. This is why IAVA has been so focused on employment initiatives, defending the new GI bill and creating a network of support among our members. Many of us have heard the tragic stories of Clay Hunt, Daniel Somers and other veterans who have died by suicide. Often these stories highlight not just the mental health challenges, but the challenges these individuals faced seeking care and obtaining VA benefits. The Suicide Prevention Office has to exist at a higher level, where it could impact both VHA and VBA. We are pleased that the Secretary has answered our call. We ask Congress to ensure that this office is fully resourced through a line-item on the budget so that it can be certain of its funding to carry out the critical mission with which it is tasked.

**The Need for Research**

[1] Office of the Inspector General, Department of Veterans Affairs. OIG Determination of Veterans Health Administration's Occupational Staffing Shortages. Washington D.C: Department of Veterans Affairs, 2015.

[2] Tanielian, Terri, Coreen Farris, Caroline Batka, Carrie M. Farmer, Eric Robinson, Charles C. Engel, Michael Robbins and Lisa H. Jaycox. Ready to Serve: Community-Based Provider Capacity to Deliver Culturally Competent, Quality Mental Health Care to Veterans and Their Families. Santa Monica, CA: RAND Corporation, 2014.

We simply don't know enough, yet, about suicide within the veteran population. We know that suicide impacts seniors disproportionately, but we don't know why. We know that the women have a high rate of suicide, but don't understand how best to intervene. We know that the post-9/11 generation is showing an increased risk, but are just starting to understand the risk factors that can really help us impact interventions. More research is critical to developing interventions. We cannot solve what we don't understand.

IAVA, and anyone serious about understanding the current state of veteran suicide, are frustrated that the Joint Suicide Data repository has not been fully utilized. That data can be critical in understanding and preventing suicide and there is no reason to not share it with the researchers and scientists outside the VA who can bring additional resources to analyzing it. Similarly, we want to see the VA's Coming Home study finally launched. Data from this study will help us to understand the transition home and define what is unique to military service from a health outcomes perspective.

A greater understanding of the unique challenges facing subgroups of vets is why IAVA supports the House-passed Female Veterans Suicide Prevention Act (H.R. 2915/S. 2487). This legislation will be critical in identifying the mental health and suicide prevention programs and services that work for women veterans. We have called on the Senate to take immediate action on the bill.

### Supporting Those Most at Risk

Finally, as a community we must provide care for those most at risk. Veterans with bad paper have a higher risk of suicide and homelessness and yet often do not have access to care. A recent report estimated there are 125,000 post-9/11 veterans with bad paper.[3] It is likely that for some, their discharge status was a result of symptoms experienced from an undiagnosed mental health injury. The current system does not make it easy to identify these individuals and get them into care. This must change. IAVA urges passage of the Fairness for Veterans? Act (S.1567/H.R.4683) as part of the solution, but we also recognize that there must be a broader solution identified through a collaborative effort between the VSO/MSO community, Congress, DoD, and VA. Suicide prevention efforts are most effective when we can identify an at risk population and provide targeted solutions to support this population. We've identified one of these populations and we know what they need. It's negligent not to take action.

In some cases, the answer might lie within the Vet Centers. This resource continues to be highly praised among IAVA's member population. We recommend a comprehensive assessment of the role the Vet Centers play in supporting veteran and family mental health. This is a critical resource and fills a specific need, particularly for veterans who may less inclined to seek services at the VA health centers, are seeking care with their family or are not eligible for VA care. We want to ensure that it is being fully utilized.

All veterans deserve the very best our nation can offer. We look forward working with you and the Administration to address these very real challenges with informed solutions.

### Statement on Receipt of Grants or Contract Funds

Neither Dr. Maffucci, nor the organization she represents, Iraq and Afghanistan Veterans of America, has received federal grant or contract funds relevant to the subject matter of this testimony during the current or past two fiscal years.

---

### Prepared Statement of Joy J. Ilem

Chairman Miller, Ranking Member Brown and Members of the Committee:

On behalf of DAV (Disabled American Veterans) and our 1.3 million members, all of whom are wartime injured or ill veterans, I am pleased to present our views at this hearing, related to the effectiveness of the mental health and suicide prevention programs of the Department of Veterans Affairs (VA), future actions that may be needed to reduce suicide among high-risk veteran populations, including women veterans and veterans who are not currently enrolled in or accessing VA services, and the progress VA has made implementing the Clay Hunt Suicide Prevention for American Veterans (SAV) Act, Public Law 114–2.

---

[3] Underserved: How the VA Wrongfully Excludes Veterans with Bad Paper. San Francisco, CA: Swords to Plowshares, 2016.

In last week's Washington Post, Harvard Psychology Professor Matthew Nock, a noted researcher on suicide, published a column worth considering on the topic before the Committee today. Professor Nock concluded in describing the present state of knowledge about suicide:

There are many well-intentioned prevention programs out there, but we have very little data on which ones work and which ones don't. .[W]e have no programs backed up by evidence from randomized controlled trials, the highest standard, showing that they stop people from ever attempting suicide. Our best bet for preventing suicide is to ramp up research and hopefully shed more light on this troubling phenomenon.

According to the Centers for Disease Control and Prevention (CDC), suicide is not a health care problem but rather, a public health and societal problem. The World Health Organization states that suicide is the 10th leading cause of death in the United States and worldwide more than 800,000 people commit suicide every year. The CDC recommends adoption of a public health model to best deal with conditions that might lead to suicidal ideation. For these reasons DAV is pleased that VA has adopted a modified public health model in its attempt to improve suicide prevention efforts in the veteran population.

Public health uses a population approach to improve health on a large scale. A population approach means focusing on prevention efforts that impact groups or populations of people as a whole, versus treatment of individuals. Second, public health focuses on preventing suicidal behavior or even ideation, before it ever occurs (primary prevention), and addresses a broad range of risk and protective factors. Third, public health holds a strong commitment to increasing understanding of suicide prevention through science, so that we can develop new and better approaches and solutions. Finally, public health values multi-disciplinary collaboration, which brings together many different perspectives and experience to strengthen the solutions for many diverse communities.

## VA Mental Health and Suicide Prevention Programs

The Vietnam War and the more recent lengthy wars in Iraq and Afghanistan have taken a toll on the mental health of the military service branches, and veterans who have returned from these operations. Combat stress and often severely disabling combat-related mental health readjustment are prevalent among Vietnam veterans and our newest generation of warfighters from Operations Enduring Freedom/Iraqi Freedom/New Dawn (OEF/OIF/OND) veterans.

Unique aspects of deployment, including the frequency and intensity of exposure to violence, injury and death, asymmetrical warfare from urban to desert to jungle environments, and suffering through or witnessing the reality of war, a truism from World War II until today, are strongly correlated with the risk of chronic post-traumatic stress disorder (PTSD) and other mental health sequalae. While veterans who served in Iraq and Afghanistan make up only a fraction of the VA patient population, they are absorbing a significant proportion of VA's specialized mental health resources. Since the wars began 15 years ago, over 2.7 million service members have deployed, more than 1.9 million are now veterans eligible for VA health care, and about 1.2 million have actually obtained VA care in some form. More than 57 percent who have received VA health care received a mental health diagnosis, prominently including PTSD. As of the end of 2015, VA was compensating nearly 830,000 veterans from all war eras for PTSD.

Applying lessons learned from prior wars, VA mounted efforts at early identification and treatment of behavioral health anomalies in enrolled OEF/OIF/OND veterans by instituting system-wide mental health screenings, adding new counseling and clinical sites, and conducting wide-scale training in evidence-based psychotherapies. While these are positive steps and VHA has made progress in disseminating knowledge about evidence-based treatment that does not guarantee implementation of such treatments. For these reasons we recommend VA collect information on the use of evidence-based psychotherapies to ensure system-wide availability of such services.

Over the past decade the VA Office of Mental Health has promoted a comprehensive set of mental health services, while VA facilities were seeing a significant increase in the number of veterans seeking care. VA has integrated a mental health presence into primary care in its Patient Aligned Care Team (PACT) model, with a goal of minimizing barriers to this specialized care, and aimed at reducing stigma. From FY 2008 to March 2014, VA provided more than 3.6 million Primary Care-Mental Health Integration (PC–MHI) clinic visits to more than 942,000 veterans. Also, VA provided specialty mental health services to more than 1.5 million veterans in fiscal year (FY) 2014.

The Government Accountability Office (GAO) and others have identified key barriers that deter veterans from seeking mental health care, including stigma, lack of understanding or awareness of the potential for improvement, lack of child care or transportation, and work or family commitments. Research shows early intervention and timely access to mental health care are key to improving quality of life, promoting recovery, obviating long-term health consequences, and minimizing the disabling effects of mental illness -and the risk for suicide.

In recent years, VA's mental health programs, including its suicide prevention efforts, have been both praised and criticized. Nevertheless, the Committee should note that VA offers an array of mental health services that is unparalleled in any other health system or individual institution in the country. The scope, depth, and breadth of VA's multivariate approaches deserve recognition. However, as noted above, VA's most significant challenge is to ensure that the dozens of developed models used in evidence-based care (many of which emerged from VA's own intramural research) are uniformly available in every Veterans Integrated Service Network-a situation that also has been criticized by both internal and external observers. Variability is the result of a number of factors including insufficient staff levels; archaic human resources operations governing personnel recruitment; availability of specialized practitioners, and lingering VA organizational and cultural challenges. DAV believes VA is making good-faith efforts to address the problems that are within its control, but Congress and the Administration need to do their part to ensure VA has the legislative authority, tools and resources to solve these specific problems.

VA increased staffing of new mental health providers following a 2012 Office of Inspector General (OIG) report on the Veterans Health Administration, titled "Review of Veterans' Access to Mental Health Care" (http://www.va.gov/oig/pubs/VAOIG–12–00900–168.pdf). In fact, VA has the highest number of mental health providers in an integrated health care system (over 5,200 employed practitioners) with specific expertise and training in post-deployment-related mental health conditions, such as PTSD. These practitioners are reinforced by investigators in VA's Research and Development Service, as well as the unique asset of the VA National Center for PTSD. VA is able to coordinate comprehensive primary and specialty care services for veterans with substance-use disorders, traumatic brain injury (TBI), and other co-occurring disorders that are tailored to meet veterans' complex health and mental health needs.

The goal of increasing staffing was to shorten waiting times for access to mental health services, and address numerous known barriers to care. However, it is unclear if all enrolled veterans are receiving the types of services they want or need-when and where they need them. Veterans, especially younger veterans, indicate they would prefer a variety of new services over medication, such as web-based life coaching and skills-building tools, intensive evidence-based therapies, as well as non-medical/non-traditional therapies, such as complementary and alternative medicine (CAM) options (i.e., yoga, meditation, acupuncture, Tai Chi). While VA is steadily increasing the availability of these new non-medical approaches, there is variability across the system related to access to CAM services.

In addition to the PACT approach, VA uses Patient-Centered Community Care (PCCC) in mental health to maximize utilization of integrated health services when enrolled veterans are unable to access direct VA care. DAV prefers VA to be the provider of these specialized services whenever possible, but immediate access to care is the most critical factor for a veteran in a mental health or emotional crisis. However, we believe VA should properly triage and make a determination for every patient based on the unique findings in each case, and develop a mental health treatment plan that meets the veteran's needs, whether in-house, in the community, or in a hybrid arrangement. A 2014 report by the RAND Corporation indicates that only 13 percent of evaluated mental health providers (not limited to VHA providers) met study criteria for readiness to provide veteran-friendly, high-quality care. According to RAND, providers working within the VHA or a military setting were more likely than others to meet the criteria, which may raise questions for some about increasing the use of non-VHA care. The report recommends conducting better assessments of civilian provider capacity, assessing the impact of trainings in cultural competency on provider capacity, expanding access to effective trainings in selected evidence-based approaches, and facilitating providers' use of evidence-based approaches.

Mr. Chairman, DAV has previously testified that, in most cases, sending veterans with war-related mental health issues out of the system is not the answer. This group can particularly benefit from VA's expertise in treating PTSD, substance-use disorders, TBI and other post-deployment transition challenges. Giving a card to a veteran with mental health challenges and leaving him or her to search for services in the community, absent VA care coordination, increases the risks for these vulnerable veterans. If veterans with mental health issues need access to care outside of the VA system, we urge VA to have routine follow-up with the veteran to ensure the patient is receiving quality care from a provider with expertise in treating veterans.

Over the years, VA has received both praise and criticism for its suicide prevention efforts and mental health services. Some veterans have undoubtedly fallen through the cracks and others have testified before Congress that VA's suicide prevention efforts were inadequate, describing barriers in access to care and the lack of time for clinicians to provide intensive evidence-based treatments for those who do access care. Veterans and family members have testified before this committee on several occasions talking about horrible failures in the system and the need to do more to ensure we do not lose another veteran to suicide. I am sure those failures weigh heavy on the many dedicated and compassionate VA mental health providers and program directors who are responsible for serving our nation's veterans. But more importantly, what can be done to ensure that any veteran who needs help gets it?

Continued evaluation of the system and a goal of continuous improvement is essential. We are pleased that VA has placed special emphasis on suicide prevention through an aggressive anti-stigma and outreach campaign, and has launched services for veterans involved in the criminal justice system. Peer Specialists, mental health consumer councils, and family and couples counseling services have also been evolving and spreading throughout VA. We have also been encouraged that VA has extended clinic hours for patients, placed VA staff on college campuses and at universities. VA's web-based self-help resources and mobile apps have been very popular and VA's coaching into care campaign focused on assisting family members and friends to get veterans the help they need has logged thousands of calls.

A 2010 progress report on the National Strategy for Suicide Prevention described the VA as "one of the most vibrant forces in the U.S. suicide prevention movement, implementing multiple levels of innovation and state of the art interventions, backed up by a robust evaluation and research capacity." More recently, Psychiatric Services, a peer-reviewed journal of the American Psychiatric Association, published a report showing that the quality of mental health care provided by VA is superior to that provided to a comparable population in the private sector.

According to the study, "in every case, VA performance was superior to that of the private sector by more than 30 percent. Compared with individuals in private plans, veterans with schizophrenia or major depression were more than twice as likely to receive appropriate initial medication treatment, and veterans with depression were more than twice as likely to receive appropriate long-term treatment." The authors concluded that "findings demonstrate the significant advantages that accrue from an organized, nationwide system of care. The much higher performance of the VA has important clinical and policy implications."

VA's current suicide prevention efforts based on a public health framework, has three major components: (1) surveillance, (2) risk and protective factors, and (3) intervention. Suicide prevention interventions aim to reduce risk factors and/or enhance protective factors that have been identified; interventions may target high-risk groups or individuals, identified based on known risk factors. Easy and quick access to care is a protective factor against suicide, and recent laws have included provisions aimed at increasing veterans' access to VA-provided or VA-funded care, including mental health care.

VA policy requires that mental health care be made available 24 hours per day in VA facilities or at local community hospitals; that new patients referred for mental health services receive an initial assessment within 24 hours and a full evaluation appointment within 14 days; and that follow-up appointments for established patients be scheduled within 30 days of initial contact. Likewise, VA has extended its care through tele-mental health capabilities so the veteran can more easily receive needed services. A full-time suicide prevention coordinator is assigned to each VA medical center and large community-based outpatient clinic. The coordinator is responsible for tracking high risk veterans (all attempters, and patients with serious suicidal ideation or others clinically determined to be at risk for suicide) as well as tracking appointments and coordinating enhanced care. The extent to which these policies are in practice broadly should continue to be a major oversight concern of this Committee. The one area we recommend VA put more focus on is crisis management. When a veteran is experiencing a mental health crisis and asking for help, there must be ready access to a mental health specialist and/or specialized program. Other areas VA should focus on include negative perceptions and concerns veterans may have about VA care, and challenges in scheduling appointments. VA should utilize its peer specialists to follow up with veterans waiting for care. According to VA, peer-to-peer interactions have been extremely helpful to the patient and treating clinicians.

In November 2011, VA launched an award-winning, national public awareness campaign called Make the Connection, which is aimed at reducing the negative perceptions associated with seeking mental health care and informing veterans, their families, friends, and members of their communities about VA resources (www.maketheconnection.net). As of July 2015, the campaign has had over 8.8 million website visits, 227,909 uses of the VA resource locator, 12 million video views, and more than 33 million Facebook comments, shares, and post likes.

The Veterans Crisis Line is another successful component in VA's suicide prevention efforts. However, despite the measurable success with answered calls, dispatched emergency services and referrals to care, service problems were identified earlier this year in a VA Office of Inspector General report. Specifically, complaints included some calls going unanswered, lack of immediate assistance, delayed arrival of emergency services, and difficulty using the call line during a crisis. Continued evaluation and program improvement is needed. For these reasons, we are pleased that an outside evaluation of the VA's mental health care system is now underway, as mandated by the Clay Hunt SAV Act, to be completed by the end of fiscal year (FY) 2017. Going forward, these evaluations will be continued on an annual basis.

Challenges also persist in suicide surveillance including timeliness of data, consistent classification of deaths as suicides, and the accuracy of information reported. Addressing these gaps is not a responsibility of VA but more so of the states' vital records agencies, coroners and medical examiners. These units of state and local government are under no federal mandate to report all suicides to any federal agency, including VA or even the CDC.

It is widely believed that inconsistent reporting of suicides across jurisdictions, as well as underreporting of suicides in general, limit the effectiveness of surveillance efforts. Classification of a death as a suicide requires a determination that death was both self-inflicted and intentional. Also, suicides may be underreported when the manner of death is misclassified as "undetermined" or "accidental" (e.g., poisonings or single-occupant automobile accidents). Additionally, each jurisdiction (state, city, Indian Tribe, or territory) governs its own rules for investigating deaths, leading to variability not only in classification but in reporting.

Based on these findings, the GAO has recommended the VA implement processes to improve the completeness, accuracy, and consistency of data reported to the VA's Behavioral Health Autopsy Program (BHAP) system, and in particular, that VA rely more on outside data sources (e.g., the DOD) to identify decedents as veterans if they are not enrolled in the agency's numerous services and benefits programs.

## High-Risk Veteran Populations Including Those Not Enrolled or Accessing VA Care, and Women Veterans

The veteran population is currently estimated at 21.7 million individuals. Of these, only 31 percent of all veterans use the VA health care system (6.7 million users). Based on this fact, it will continue to be a challenge for VA to provide successful outreach to veterans that do not use VA but who may need VA's specialized mental health services. There have been several examples highlighted in the media about military units that have suffered losses to suicide without veterans getting any help in the VA or in the private sector. This past weekend, to contribute to the ongoing suicide prevention efforts for our nation's veterans, DAV along with a coalition of non-profits sponsored a "Spartan Weekend" for ill and injured veterans, which centered on the promise that they would not take their own life without reaching out to someone for help. The goal is to help isolated veterans reconnect with their battle buddy, unit members and other veterans who may need care. The event reached 1.8 million Facebook and other social media users and resulted in a number of veterans reaching out for help.

Meeting the unique needs of women veterans has been a priority for DAV. According to VA, over the past decade, there has been a 154 percent increase in the number of women veterans accessing VHA mental health services. Women veterans comprise 9 percent of the total veteran population but constitute the fastest growing veteran sub-population. Since 2000, the number of women veterans using VA health care has more than doubled. VA offers a comprehensive array of mental health and specialized post-deployment mental health services to women and VA's Uniform Mental Health Services Handbook requires that mental health services be provided as needed to women veterans at an equivalent level to that of their male counterparts system-wide, and that providers be capable and competent to meet the unique needs of women.

VA conducts annual, comprehensive assessments of suicide deaths that occur among veterans using VA health services. These assessments evaluate gender differences in suicide rates. According to VA, suicide rates among women veterans have increased in recent years, yet are lower than suicide rates among male veterans. VA continues to conduct important research to identify risk factors and patterns of suicide in veterans, including those that may be linked to gender. In one recent study, VA researchers found rates of suicide to be higher among women who report having experienced military sexual trauma (MST), contrasted with those who did not.

VA partnered with 23 states to report information from death certificates on veteran deaths by suicide to learn more about patterns and rates. Recently, this effort allowed VA researchers to evaluate preliminary estimates of suicide rates, including those who do and those who do not use VA health care services. These estimates were based on information for the years 2000 through 2010 and include gender-specific information, including:

- Suicide rates were nearly six times higher in women veterans than in civilian women.
- Suicide among all women veterans was 34.6 per 100,000 in 2010. This rate increased 40 percent since 2000, from 24.7 per 100,000.
- The suicide rate among male veterans was 36 per 100,000.

In 2010, women veterans who used VA health services were 75 percent less likely to die by suicide than women veterans who did not use VA health services. This data suggests that VA's mental health programs for women, including suicide prevention efforts, are showing a positive impact. VA also found that for women veterans, there is a greater likelihood of using firearms as the method of suicide, (i.e., women veterans who die by suicide are 18 percent more likely than civilian women to use firearms as the instrument of death). Furthermore, the firearm suicide rate among women veterans has increased faster and to a greater degree than suicide rates among women veterans using other methods. This type of gender-specific data collection can aid VA in improving mental health services for our women veterans.

As documented in DAV's 2014 report, Women Veterans: the Long Journey Home, women's military and wartime deployment experiences and reintegration processes are inherently different from those of their male counterparts. Research indicates that both men and women may develop PTSD as a response to combat exposure, but women are more likely to manifest depression as a co-occurring disorder. Women are less likely than men to display anger and resort to substance use. Women are more likely to develop depression, or an eating or anxiety disorder, but without a diagnosis of PTSD. Findings also show that when women return from deployment, the camaraderie and support from their male peers is often short-lived, resulting in isolation for many. Studies have shown that peer support is important to a successful transition, but women report they often cannot find a network of women who can relate to their military or wartime service.

While VA is recognized for its longstanding expertise in specialized mental health and post-deployment mental health services, it has struggled to establish system-wide access to gender-specific group counseling, residential treatment, and specialty inpatient programs to serve women. Improved access to these programs is essential for recovery and effective reintegration, therefore VA must ensure all outpatient and residential programs have environments that can accommodate women with safety, privacy, and respect. Existing programs should be re-evaluated to ensure they are appropriately tailored to meet the unique mental health care and post-deployment transition challenges women experience in serving in war.

### Update on the Clay Hunt SAV Act, Public Law 114–2

The Clay Hunt Suicide Prevention for American Veterans (SAV) Act included provisions to:

- Extend for one year the existing five-year post-discharge period of open eligibility for VA health care for combat veterans covering illnesses that have not been medically proven to be related to their military service;
- Increase access to mental health care by creating a peer support and community outreach pilot program including an interactive website of available resources;
- Create a pilot program to repay loan debt of psychiatry students for VA recruitment purposes; and
- Conduct an annual evaluation of VA mental health and suicide prevention program.

Based on our understanding, VA is still working to implement most of the provisions in the Clay Hunt SAV Act. The VISNs have been chosen for establishing a community peer outreach network, developing website resources is in progress, the educational loan language is still pending in the regulatory process and the RFP or Request for Proposals for the Independent Evaluation has gone out.

## DAV Recommendations

- DAV urges Congress and the Administration to ensure ample resources are provided for VA mental health programs, including comprehensive treatment for serious mental illness and sexual trauma, readjustment counseling, peer-to-peer programs, promotion of evidence-based treatments for post-traumatic stress disorder, and specialty substance-use disorder services to provide effective mental health care for all veterans needing such services.
- VA should continually strive to improve access and services for veterans in crisis and those seeking VA primary mental health care and specialized programs. VA should continue its targeted outreach, anti-stigma, and early intervention efforts, and routine screening for new veterans returning from wartime deployments.
- VA should continue research in mental health to study gaps in care and develop best practices in screening, diagnosis, and treatment for post-deployment readjustment, as well as studies focused on understanding and reducing suicide in the veteran population.
- VA should conduct health services research on effective stigma reduction, differences in gender readjustment, suicide prevention, and treatment of acute co-occurring PTSD, mild traumatic brain injury, and substance-use disorders in combat veterans.
- VA should increase innovative programs such as telehealth for increasing access to gender-sensitive mental health treatment programs for women veterans.
- VA should develop a standardized approach to transition women with serious mental health deficits, including those who have experienced sexual assault, from DOD to VA care.
- Congress should expand the authority for the VA Readjustment Counseling Service's women veterans retreat program. The VA Office of Research and Development should study the program to determine its key success factors, its effectiveness as an alternative treatment regimen, and whether it can be replicated in other settings.

## Closing

Despite obvious improvements, it is clear that more progress needs to be achieved by VA to fulfill the nation's obligations to veterans who are challenged by serious and, in some cases, chronic mental illness-particularly in all eras of war veterans, including younger veterans who are confronted by post-deployment repatriation and transition challenges. Currently, there is a pressing need for timely access to mental health services for many returning injured and ill veterans, particularly in early intervention services for veterans with substance-use disorders, and for evidence-based treatments for those with PTSD, suicidal ideation, depression and other consequences of combat exposure. If these symptoms are not readily addressed at onset, they can easily compound and become chronic and lifelong. Delays or failures in addressing these problems can result in risky behavior, job and family disintegration, incarceration, homelessness, and suicide.

DAV appreciates the efforts made by VA to improve the safety, consistency, and effectiveness of mental health care programs for all veterans. We urge VA to continue research on suicide prevention efforts and finding innovative ways to engage all veterans. We also appreciate that Congress continues to provide funding to VA in pursuit of a comprehensive set of services to meet the mental health needs of veterans, in particular veterans with wartime service who present post-deployment readjustment needs. To this end, we urge the Committee's continued oversight of VA's progress in fully implementing its Mental Health Strategic Plan.

Chairman Miller and Members of the Committee, this concludes my statement. DAV appreciates the opportunity to provide this testimony, and I would be pleased to address any of the topics discussed in this statement.

---

### Prepared Statement of Thomas J. Berger, Ph.D.

Chairman Miller, Ranking Member Brown, and Distinguished Members of the House Veterans Affairs Committee, Vietnam Veterans of America (VVA) thanks you for the opportunity to present our testimony regarding the Department of Veterans Affairs (VA) efforts to reduce suicide among the veteran population. We should also like to thank you for your overall concern about the mental health care of our troops and veterans.

The timing of this HVAC hearing is particularly important as a recent National Center for Health Statistics report found that suicide in the United States has surged to the highest levels in nearly 30 years, with increases in every age group except older adults (i.e., declining for only one age group: men and women over 75). The rise was particularly steep for women where the suicide rate for middle-aged women, ages 45 to 64, jumped by 63 percent over the period of the study, while it rose by 43 percent for men in that age range, the sharpest increase for males of any age. It was also substantial among middle-aged Americans, whose suicide rates had been stable or falling since the 1950s. The overall suicide rate rose by 24 percent from 1999 to 2014, according to the report, and the increases were so widespread that they lifted the nation's suicide rate to 13 per 100,000 people, the highest since 1986. There is absolutely no doubt that this country is in the midst of a public health crisis with suicide.

Nowhere is this more true than in the veterans community as we learned back in February 2013 from the VA's report on veterans who die by suicide. This report painted a shocking portrait of what's happening among our older vets (see chart below) ——

| Age group | Non-veteran | Veteran |
| --- | --- | --- |
| 29 and younger | 24.4% | 5.8% |
| 30-39 | 20.0 | 8.9 |
| 40-49 | 23.5 | 15.0 |
| 50-59 | 16.9 | 20.0 |
| 60-69 | 7.4 | 16.8 |
| 70-79 | 4.2 | 19.0 |
| 80 and older | 3.6 | 14.5 |

**Almost three-quarters of veterans who commit suicide are age 50 or older according to this report.**

And even though suicide has become a major issue for the military over the last decade, most research by the Pentagon and the Veterans Affairs Department has focused on men, who account for more than 90% of the nation's 22 million former troops. Little has been known about female veteran suicide until recently.

According to an LA Times article in July 2016, the suicide rates are highest among young female veterans—for women ages 18 to 29, veterans kill themselves at nearly 12 times the rate of nonveterans. And, according to the Times same article, among the cohort of nearly 174,000 veteran suicides in 21 states between 2000 and 2010, the suicide rate of female vets closely approximates that of male counterparts—i.e., women vets 28.7 per 100,000 vs 32.1 per 100, 000 male vets.

However, we must not forget that it is from the VA's 2013 report noted above that the figure of 22 veteran suicides per day is calculated. This number is suspect because the data only represent numbers reported from 21 states from 1999 through 2011 and did not include states with massive veteran communities, like California and Texas which didn't report suicides to the VA at that time.

If the media are going to focus on this number, they need to make sure that they are targeting the right generation because according to the report, the majority of veteran suicides are committed by Vietnam-era veterans, yet the media is surprisingly quiet on this point. Therefore, VVA calls for an updated veteran suicide report that includes data from all 50 states and U.S. territories, and also strongly suggests that VA mental health services develop a nationwide strategy to address the problem of suicides among our older veterans - particularly Vietnam-era veterans. To do so, the VA should seriously consider the establishment of an Advisory Board of key VA stakeholders involved in suicide prevention, education, treatment, and research.

VVA understands that it is very challenging to determine an exact number of suicides. Some troops who return from deployment become stronger from having survived their experiences. Too many others are wracked by memories of what they have experienced. This translates into extreme issues and risk-taking behaviors when they return home, which is one of the reasons why veteran suicides have attracted so much attention in the media. Many times, suicides are not reported, and it can be very difficult to determine whether or not a particular individual's death was intentional. For a suicide to be recognized, examiners must be able to say that the deceased meant to die. Other factors that contribute to the difficulty are differences among states as to who is mandated to report a death, as well as changes over time in the coding of mortality data. Nevertheless, according to the American Foundation for Suicide Prevention, in more than 120 studies of a series of completed suicides, at least 90 percent of the individuals involved were suffering from a mental illness at the time of their death. The most important interventions are recognizing and treating these underlying illnesses, such as depression, alcohol and substance abuse, post-traumatic stress disorder and traumatic brain injury. Many veterans (and active duty military) resist seeking help because of the stigma associated with mental illness, or they are unaware of the warning signs and treatment options. These barriers must be identified and overcome.

To be fair, VVA recognizes that over the past year, the VA has developed a number of strategies to reduce suicides and suicide behaviors in the veterans' community since HVAC's Oversight Subcommittee July 2010 hearing entitled "Examining the Progress of Suicide Prevention Outreach Efforts at the VA". These efforts have included a February 2016 announcement that improvements to enhance and accelerate progress at the Veterans Crisis Line were made by moving the Veterans Crisis Line into VA's Member Services under a director with extensive clinical social work background, and that by the end of this year, every veteran in crisis will have their call promptly answered by an experienced VA responder. That will mean non-core calls will be directed appropriately to other VA entities that can best address their questions or concerns and presumably, will eliminate the hundreds of "dropped" calls we have all read about. VA also committed to increase staff at the Veterans Crisis Line Center.

Then on March 8, the VA also publicly announced changes to be made to its suicide prevention programs, including:

1. Elevating VA's suicide-prevention program with additional resources to manage and strengthen current programs and initiatives;

2. Meeting urgent mental health needs by providing veterans with the goal of same-day evaluations and access by the end of calendar year 2016;

3. Establishing a new standard of care by using measures of veteran-reported symptoms to tailor mental health treatments to individual needs;

4. Launching a new study, "Coming Home from Afghanistan and Iraq," to look at the impact of deployment and combat as it relates to suicide, mental health, and well-being;

5. Using predictive modeling to guide early interventions for suicide prevention;

6. Using data on suicide attempts and overdoses to guide strategies to prevent suicide;

7. Increasing the availability of naloxone rescue kits throughout VA to prevent deaths from opioid overdoses;

8. Enhancing veteran mental health access by establishing three regional telemental health hubs; and

9. Continuing to partner with the DoD on suicide prevention and other efforts for a seamless transition from military service to civilian life.

While these initiatives are laudable, VVA also believes strongly that they cannot fully succeed without a significant increase in the recruitment, hiring, and retention of VA mental health staff, as well as timely access to VA mental health clinical facilities and programs, especially for our rural veterans. This committee must ensure that our veterans and their families are given access to the resources and programs necessary to stem the tide of veteran suicide.

Once again, on behalf of VVA's National Officers, Board, and general membership, thank you for your leadership in holding this important hearing on a topic that is literally of vital interest to so many veterans, and should be of keen interest to all Americans who care about our nation's veterans. I shall be glad to answer any questions.

## VIETNAM VETERANS OF AMERICA

### Funding Statement

### May 12, 2016

The national organization Vietnam Veterans of America (VVA) is a non-profit veterans' membership organization registered as a 501(c)(19) with the Internal Revenue Service. VVA is also appropriately registered with the Secretary of the Senate and the Clerk of the House of Representatives in compliance with the Lobbying Disclosure Act of 1995.

VVA is not currently in receipt of any federal grant or contract, other than the routine allocation of office space and associated resources in VA Regional Offices for outreach and direct services through its Veterans Benefits Program (Service Representatives). This is also true of the previous two fiscal years.

For Further Information, Contact:
Executive Director for Policy and Government Affairs
Vietnam Veterans of America.
(301) 585–4000, extension 127

---

### Prepared Statement of Kim Ruocco

Tragedy Assistance Program for Survivors (TAPS) is the national organization providing compassionate care for the families of America's fallen military heroes. TAPS provides peer-based emotional support, grief and trauma resources, grief seminars and retreats for adults, 'Good Grief Camps' for children, case work assistance, connections to community-based care, and a 24/7 resource and information helpline for all who have been affected by a death in the Armed Forces. Services are provided to families at no cost to them. We do all of this without financial support from the Department of Defense. TAPS is funded by the generosity of the American people.

TAPS was founded in 1994 by Bonnie Carroll following the death of her husband in a military plane crash in Alaska in 1992. Since then, TAPS has offered comfort and care to more than 50,000 bereaved surviving family members. For more information, please visit www.TAPS.org

TAPS currently receives no government grants or funding.

### Kim Ruocco

Kim Ruocco is presently the Chief External Relations Officer for Suicide Prevention and Postvention for the Tragedy Assistance Program for Survivors (TAPS). Ms. Ruocco is an international public speaker who has a unique combination of personal and professional experience, education and training that provides a comprehensive understanding of suicide prevention and postvention. Ms. Ruocco has been the keynote speaker at many national events, most notably the Department of Defense (DOD)/Department of Veterans'Affairs(VA) Suicide Prevention Conference, VA Suicide Prevention Month, The LOSS team conference, AAS/AFSP Healing Conference, IAVA Clay Hunt announcement and multiple USMC, Army, ANG and Navy safety stand downs. She has appeared in multiple media outlets including CNN, Fox News, Al Jazeera, NPR and NBC radio. She has been the topic of many magazine articles including Men's Health, Christian Science Monitor, Stars and Stripes and Marine Times. Ms. Ruocco is regularly quoted in national newspapers articles on the topics of Suicide, Military Culture, Mental Illness, PTSD and VA and DOD policy matters.

Ms. Ruocco has been instrumental in raising awareness using the voices of military suicide survivors. She developed suicide survivor panels that testified in multiple venues including the DOD/VA suicide prevention task force, National Action Alliance and DOD/VA conferences. She assisted in the development of the Department of Defense Suicide prevention Office (DSPO) Postvention Toolkit, and was a reviewer for the current national strategy for postvention. Ms. Ruocco assisted in the development of the USMC's "Never Leave a Marine Behind" program and is a participant in the training video. She was the Family Liaison Contact for the USMC/AAS psychological autopsy research project that provided key prevention information for the USMC. She and her sons are also lead participants in the Sesame Street "When Families Grieve" video which is distributed internationally to families who have a recent death. Ms. Ruocco regularly briefs the DSPO and Navy on the family perspective of risk factors and gaps in service. She has also testified before the Senate Committee on Veterans' Affairs and is considered a subject matter expert for suicide pre and postvention.

Ms. Ruocco has developed comprehensive, peer-based programs that offer comfort and care to all those who are grieving the loss of a service member to suicide. She created a team of peer-professionals who provide care and comfort to nearly 5000 survivors of military suicide. The most impactful of these services is the TAPS Annual Survivors of Suicide Loss Seminar, which offers hope and healing to thousands of survivors, and provides a camp and military mentoring for the children of the fallen. Her programming has been ground breaking in the field of postvention and has been incorporated into many civilian postvention programs.

Ms. Ruocco is currently the co-lead on the National Action Alliance Military and Family Task force and a member of the National Expert Advisory Panel for Research.

Ms. Ruocco holds a BA in Human Services and Psychology from the University of Massachusetts and a Masters degree in Clinical Social Work from Boston University. She is also the surviving widow of Marine Corp Major John Ruocco, who died by suicide in 2005.

Chairman Miller, Ranking Member Brown, and other distinguished members of the Veterans Affairs Committee, the Tragedy Assistance Program for Survivors (TAPS) thanks you for the opportunity to share the stories of surviving family members of service members and veterans who have completed suicide and to offer suggestions on how to prevent other families from suffering the same tragedy. We are appreciative of the work this subcommittee has done in the past to improve benefits for the survivors of those who have made the greatest sacrifice for our country.

**How TAPS Helps Survivors**

The Tragedy Assistance program for Survivors (TAPS) is a national organization providing compassionate care for the families of America's fallen military heroes. TAPS provides peer-based emotional support, grief and trauma resources, grief seminars and retreats for adults, "Good Grief Camps" for children, casework assistance, connections to community-based care, and 24/7 resource and information helpline for all who have been affected by a death in the Armed Forces. Services are provided to families and battle buddies at no cost to them. TAPS does all of this without financial support from the Department of Defense (DoD or the Department of Veterans' Affairs (VA). TAPS is funded by the generosity of the American people

Bonnie Carroll, following the death of her husband in a military plane crash in Alaska in 1992 founded TAPS. Since then, TAPS has offered comfort and care to more than 50,000 bereaved family members worldwide.

**TAPS Special Care for the Survivors Whose Loved Ones Complete Suicide**

My name is Kim Ruocco and I came to TAPS seeking support in 2006 following the death of my husband, Marine Corp Major John Ruocco. John died by suicide after suffering for years with untreated depression and PTSD. He was an attack helicopter pilot who flew 75 combat missions in Iraq and died three months after he returned. When John died, I was overcome with emotions and questions. I was desperate to talk to others who had experienced this kind of loss. I had a lot of questions like "How do I tell my two boys, who were 8 and 10, that their Dad made it safely back from combat and then took his own life?" I had questions about spirituality and increased risk for my children and myself and a need to know why someone dies by suicide. I realized that a death by suicide required a different kind of grief journey than other military deaths.

In 2007 Bonnie Carroll and I developed a comprehensive Suicide Loss Survivor Program. The program is divided into three parts:

- POSTVENTION-postvention is prevention. Those who are exposed to suicide, especially those who were intimately connected to the deceased, are at higher risk of suicide themselves. Postvention is an intervention that provides care to all those who are grieving a death by suicide in hopes of decreasing risk and providing a path to healing. TAPS has developed a program that allows peer professionals to connect immediately with new survivors. New survivors are offered peer based support, resources and referrals to trauma care and seminars designed specifically for healing after suicide.

- INTERVENTION-survivors of traumatic loss are at increased risk for suicide, mental health disorders and addiction. Whether killed in action, illness, accident or suicide, survivors may be at risk for suicide. TAPS staff is trained in Applied Suicide Intervention Skills Training (ASIST). This training allows our staff to identify those at risk and connect them with the care they need.
- PREVENTION-with each suicide comes a story of a service member or veteran who did not survive his or her injury or illness. These stories provide us with an extraordinary amount of information that can be used in prevention efforts. TAPS has been the voice of suicide survivors for over a decade. Information from our survivors has informed policy and protocols for each of the services as well as the DOD and VA. We are grateful to be asked once again to testify on behalf of these surviving families.

### Surviving Family Members of Military Suicide Share Their Stories

One of the largest growing populations in our TAPS family is our surviving families of military suicide. TAPS presently has over 7000 suicide loss survivors and 700 survivors of murder-suicide. We average 3 to 4 new suicide survivors everyday.

For the purpose of today's hearing, I would like to focus on the suicide loss population within TAPS. Survivors of military suicide hold a wealth of information on the multiple factors that lead up to a death by suicide. They are on the front lines of a service member's or veteran's battle with PTSD, mental illness, moral injury and the multiple stressors associated with military life. They are witness to the challenges of stigma associated with mental health and the barriers to care for those who are suffering. Survivors of veteran suicide loss can provide us with a picture of the potential impact of challenges within the VA system. Today's testimony is a summary of information gathered from our survivors' journeys. I have narrowed it down to two prominent and consistent themes.

### Barriers To Care

We know from research that treatment works and that those who are in the care of the VA have a lower rate of suicide. In each case of a TAPS family whose loved one died by suicide, the veteran was not enrolled in a consistent, effective, evidence based treatment at the VA. In most cases the veteran struggled to get the care they needed in a timely fashion. In some cases the veteran himself became the first barrier to good care because of their cultural beliefs and stigma regarding mental health. This reluctance to share their true story, in combination with institutional barriers, can become the perfect storm for a veteran who is suffering. Families of these veterans struggled to help their loved one and often became frustrated and overwhelmed with navigating the system. Many of them expressed frustration with the lack of their involvement in assessment and treatment. They claim that part of the veteran culture is to not complain or admit to emotional or physical pain and to downplay how serious the issues actually are. Families feel strongly that if they were present for intakes and evaluations there would have been a more accurate diagnosis and treatment plan. Additionally these families long for a network of peer support where they could share information ideas about what helped and offer support to one another.

Here are some stories from TAPS families whose service member or veteran faced barriers to care:

### PCS Edward Michael Gilkes

"Eddie", was stationed at Ft Benning Ga. training to be an Airborne soldier. Just before graduation he was accidently blown up by a claymore mine. He spent two years in and out of Army hospitals trying to recover from debilitating migraine headaches, blurred vision, ringing in his ears and nausea. Despite his pain and multiple doctor visits, Eddie never gave up trying to reach his dreams. He attempted to complete Ranger training three times but in each case he failed due to his ongoing medical issues.

In May of 2012, Eddie was honorably discharged from the Army following a medical board review. He was not given a disability rating or sequential pay. Eddie moved in with his parents because he could not afford to live on his own. He spent one year waiting to be assessed for care by the VA. During this time he was riddled with pain and started to lose hope that he would ever get better. When his assessment was complete, Edward waited another 6 months for an appointment with the doctor. At the appointment he was given painkillers, a brain scan and was told to come back in 3 months. Edward returned in 3 months and waited all day in the waiting room. At the end of the day he was told that he would have to reschedule because there was no longer time to see him. The next appointment he could get was 2 months away.

During this period Edward was also waiting for a disability rating from the VA. His diagnosis was TBI and PTSD along with chronic pain related to the training accident. Despite documentation of all these conditions, disability was denied with one of the reasons being that he "had not had enough visits with the VA." Eddie became so frustrated and hopeless that he gave up trying to get care from the VA. He began looking for a job and was hired to work on the pipeline. This work was very difficult for him. He had to take frequent breaks because of his pain and he had difficulty concentrating. Co-workers often had to cover for him. After a little over a year, he was laid off. Eddie moved in with his brother and applied for unemployment but his spirit was broken. On October 26th, 2015 PCS Edward Michael Gilkes died by suicide. He left a note saying "I have no purpose in life."

### CPL Kevin Schranz

Kevin was a Marine Corp machine gunner who served two combat tours in Afghanistan. During his second tour he received a couple of minor injuries from explosions. He experienced ringing in his ears and a minor eye injury that could develop into a more significant injury in the future. He was honorably discharged in 2014. He and his wife moved to Connecticut where he enrolled in college and he tried to transition to the civilian world. During this time Kevin began to have some anxiety and sleep problems. He told his wife that he had seen some "intense things" and couldn't get them out of his mind. Kevin started counseling at the Vet Center and put in a VA claim for his eye injury, tinnitus and anxiety.

Kevin's wife, Abby says her husband became more anxious and paranoid. He started to be afraid to be alone and carried his gun with him. She encouraged him to go to the VA and be assessed for PTSD. Abby says that her husband "trusted the system" and was anxious to find out "what was wrong with him." Kevin did go to the VA and was tested for PTSD. Months later Kevin was denied benefits for his eye injury and was told that he did not have PTSD. This finding was devastating to Kevin. He said to his wife that this was just a problem with him. He wrote a letter to his wife stating that everyone would be better off without him. He also left a suicide note that said, in part "This is my own fault, this is not a PTSD problem so please do not politicize it." Abby looked at his records, after he died, and was surprised to see that he denied many of the issues that she witnessed him having, such as driving recklessly. Abby expressed regret that she was not involved in the assessment. She also wished her husband was immediately enrolled in the VA and given treatment for his combat exposure without having to "prove" he was sick.

### Sgt. Raymond Burnside

Ray was a Special Ops medic for the Army. He had one tour in Iraq and another in Afghanistan. Ray enlisted right out of high school when he was just 18 years old. He was determined to do something important with his life and also wanted to avoid ending up like his Dad, who was a veteran who died by suicide in the early 90s. Ray was honorably discharged from the Army in 2012. He claimed that he was fine and did not need help with the things he had seen and done in combat. His mom was concerned because she could see that he was drinking a lot and seemed to isolate himself frequently. Ray started school but found it very challenging. He would tell his Mom that no one understood him and he would get really angry at things the professors would say. He seemed more and more agitated and angry and his drinking increased. He dropped out of school and went on what his mom described as "a quest to fit in and calm his emotions." At one point he disappeared saying he was going to join the French foreign legion. He came back weeks later saying that he was so drunk that he lost his way. His friends and family became very concerned about him. They asked if he might be suffering from PTSD and he would respond, "No, I am just a loser, it is all my fault."

In July of 2014 Ray was finally convinced to go to the VA. He went by himself saying, "I can handle it." Ray returned home, after his first visit, enraged. He said that they treated him like he was just trying to get attention. He said that he was told that he is not as bad as other guys they had seen. Ray told his family that this is exactly what he feared that he wouldn't be believed and that people would think he is weak and making up his symptoms. His family felt helpless. They wondered if Ray had shared just how bad his symptoms were because he had so much shame about them. For the next couple of years Ray would self-medicate with alcohol and periodically become suicidal. His mom would call the VA asking for help and didn't know how to get the help her son needed. Once she was able to get him committed to inpatient care but he left after three days saying he couldn't "be confined like that because it brought him back to a place he didn't want to go." The day before Ray died he cut his wrist very badly. His Mom found him trying to stitch it closed by himself. She convinced him to go to the ER only by convincing him that they could tell the hospital that he cut his arm on a broken window. They went to the VA emergency room and he was stitched up and released. He went home and began drinking. By the next day he was saying that he was going to kill himself. His mom was desperate to save him and was able to convince him to get in the car with her. Unfortunately at a stop sign he jumped out of the car and ran. He was found hours later, hanging in a hotel room.

## PEER–BASED SUPPORT

In each case the family tells TAPS that their veteran only wanted to talk to someone who has "been there." The veteran had shame and guilt about the symptoms they were feeling and thought these symptoms were a weakness in them, not an illness. This false belief became a barrier to getting a good assessment and to finding appropriate treatment and staying in treatment. Peer support can be used to build trust that eventually leads to an understanding that their symptoms are real and valid and that there is treatment available that works. Peers serve as a beacon of hope for those who are struggle and can offer a road map on navigating the system.

The Fisher family shared their thoughts about how peer-based support could have helped their son Fritz.

### Fritz Fisher

Fritz Fisher was a Marine veteran who had served two tours in Iraq and was honorably discharged from the Marine Corp in 2004. Fritz was a field operator in Iraq and had to leave mid tour because his commitment was up. He married Amanda soon after discharge from the Marines. Within days of his discharge he experienced extreme guilt for leaving his buddies in a war zone and had nightmares and flashbacks related to his tour. Amanda encouraged him to go the VA and get assessed. At first he refused saying, "I need to suck it up" and "it wouldn't look good." Fritz resisted care and at the same time his symptoms continued to escalate. He was having angry outbursts and panic attacks. He self-medicated with alcohol which just increased his problems. Finally Amanda was able to convince him to go to the VA. According to Amanda, it took two years for Fritz to get a PTSD disability rating of 30% and many months to see a doctor. When he finally saw the doctor, he was given medication and not offered counseling for his emotional pain and PTSD. Fritz dropped out of treatment telling his wife that it wasn't helping and he didn't feel better. In 2010 Fritz became a government contractor and deployed back to Iraq. He told his wife that this would help him and that it is where he feels most comfortable. In 2011 Fitz returned from Iraq and started having problems. He had chest pain and panic attacks. He was drinking and smoking marijuana to ease his symptoms. He didn't want to go back to the VA because "he didn't just want to be drugged like my buddies." Amanda was desperate to help him but didn't know how. Their life became a cycle of anxiety, angry outbursts, addiction and crisis. When Fritz was in crisis Amanda would take him to the VA ER. She states that many times they would wait all day and sometimes not get an appointment. On several occasions Fritz stormed out yelling "no one gives a shit." In 2012 Fritz had hit rock bottom. He had started huffing air dust. He became suicidal and called his parents. His parents drove and picked him up. They also did not know how to help him so they drove him to the VA. They were told they would see him when they could fit him in. They waited for several hours and Fritz stormed out. Fritz only tried to get treatment one more time before his death. He went to a civilian, mental health provider and they told him that he needed to go to the VA. Fritz over-dosed on air dust on October 2, 2014. His wife wishes that her husband had more peer support to encourage treatment and normalize his symptoms. She also wishes she had a place to get answers on how to help him.

A veteran recently told me "I was homeless and living out of my truck when I met my peer support specialist 3 years ago. He helped me in all areas of my life and I am proud to say that tomorrow I am closing on a home."

### Recommendations

1.Increase number of mental health care providers who are trained in evidence based best practice for treatment of injuries and illnesses related to these conflicts. At each contact a veteran should be able to get appropriate mental health care in a timely manner. This is especially crucial for entry points during crisis, such as emergency rooms and outpatient clinics.

2.Develop family advocacy and information groups that can offer support and guidance to those who are supporting a veteran.

3.Develop an avenue for family members to call for professional advice on how to help their loved one.

4.Make peer support specialist a line item. Peer support is an invaluable tool and a reciprocal relationship that adds value to all involved. Peer support specialist can be used to reach out to veterans where they are and build a bridge toward the professional mental health care they need. Peer professionals can be used in numerous impactful ways including navigating paper work, running support groups, normalizing symptoms and validating that treatment works.

5.Increase incentives for and streamline process for becoming a peer mental health professional. In the field of social work we often say "there is no better clinician than one who has personal experience and professional training". In the case of veterans, personal experience adds a level of trust and credibility that greatly increases the probability of a veteran seeking treatment and staying in treatment.

We hope you will consider our recommendations as you consider the ways that the Department of Veterans Affairs can reach out and help those veterans who are contemplating suicide. Our families shared their stories so that all may learn and identify what brought their loved one to take their lives. TAPS stands ready to work with you to end this national epidemic.

---

### Prepared Statement of Dr. Maureen McCarthy

Good morning, Chairman Miller, Ranking Member Brown, and members of the Committee. Thank you for the opportunity to discuss the effectiveness of the Department of Veterans Affairs (VA) mental health programs. I am accompanied by Dr. Harold Kudler, Chief Consultant, Mental Health Services, and Dr. Caitlin Thompson, National Director, Suicide Prevention, Veterans Health Administration.

VA has developed the largest integrated suicide prevention program in the country. We have over 800 dedicated and passionate employees, including Suicide Prevention Coordinators, Veterans Crisis Line staff, epidemiologists, and researchers, who spend each and every day solely working on suicide prevention efforts and care for our Veterans. Our overarching strategy is based on enhancing Veterans' access to high-quality mental health care and implementing upstream programs designed to help prevent Veterans from even considering suicide. Losing one Veteran to suicide shatters an entire world. Veterans who reach out for help must receive that help when and where they need it in terms that they value.

### Preventing Veterans Suicide - A Call to Action

The Department of Veterans Affairs (VA) hosted a summit on "Preventing Veterans Suicide - A Call to Action" on February 2, 2016, to bring together Veterans, families, other Federal agencies, community providers, subject matter experts, and other key partners to enhance our work on suicide prevention. VA continues to partner with more than 150 non-Federal mental health organizations around suicide prevention. Alongside these partners, we remain strongly committed to preventing Veteran suicide. We recognize that we can't do this alone, and we continue to develop and prioritize these partnerships.

Powerful for so many attendees were the stories shared both by Veterans and by families. The families of Clay Hunt and Daniel Somers have testified before this committee with us several years ago. What they shared then and in other settings and again at our Call to Action truly has been an extremely powerful and compelling message to us. We see them and other families as essential partners to help us continue to think through and develop our services.

In addition, we heard from two extraordinary Veterans, Mr. John Heitzman and Mr. Brent Rice, during the Call to Action. They told their stories of falling into significant crises and seriously considering suicide. They then spoke about the power of connecting with VA Suicide Prevention Coordinators and VA clinicians who were integral in helping them to recover and lead fulfilling and healthy lives. All these stories were videotaped and are available through the following links: Veteran - John Heitzman - YouTube and Veteran- Brent Rice - YouTube

The message from these Veterans was one that truly resonated with us. Just as preventing death from heart attacks does not begin in the Intensive Care Unit, likewise suicide prevention does not necessarily begin with our Crisis Line or our interventions when suicide is imminent. Instead, it's about finding hope, leading a high-quality life, developing strong, meaningful relationships, and celebrating our reasons for living. Engaging Veterans in VA care, and particularly in our whole system of care, is a key part of prevention. Also engagement with communities is essential.

Just like preventing death from heart disease involves our efforts in promoting healthy living, addressing risk factors, intervening when blood pressure or lipid profiles signal problems, there are precursor steps we continue to take to prevent suicide. Focusing on the social aspects of Veterans lives, working to advocate for their benefits, to assist them with jobs and functioning in those jobs, screening for signs of depression to include screening for substance use disorders, Post-traumatic Stress Disorder which is strongly associated with substance use and dependence, Military Sexual Trauma, and Intimate Partner Violence, intervening with our Justice Outreach System, preventing homelessness, and providing a system of medical care for Veterans,—all of these are significant interventions in VA which are part of our comprehensive suicide prevention program. That is the message these two Veterans who spoke so eloquently communicated.

The summit generated a series of very clear recommendations for VA. One frequently voiced recommendation was for VA and the Department of Defense (DoD) to partner on improving the transition from military service to civilian life. This builds upon the Presidential Executive Action of August 26, 2014, requiring DoD to automatically enroll all service members identified as having a mental health problem into DoD's inTransition program and, upon separation from the military, provide a warm handoff to VA care or community care. Research demonstrates that the time of transition out of military service is a time of significant stress and increased health risk for service members and their families. This includes being a time of increased risk for suicide.

VA research has indicated that rates of suicide among those who use VA services have not shown increases similar to those observed in all Veterans and the general U.S. population. This research suggests that an improved healthcare transition between DoD and VA could help mitigate suicide risk as well as other increased risks of morbidity. Focusing on this transition would advance the Departments to a proactive population health approach focused on prevention through early engagement. To accomplish this, VA must facilitate transitioning service members' enrollment in VA health care.

The Call to Action summit generated multiple additional recommendations and initiatives to strengthen VA's approach to Suicide Prevention. Significantly, a pilot project is underway to evaluate risk intervention strategies based on data that predict who would be at risk for suicide before these individuals reach a crisis. Also, VA continues to actively monitor suicide related behaviors through the Suicide Prevention Applications Network (SPAN). We are working to develop a dashboard that will allow ongoing surveillance to support the identification of possible clusters of suicide-related behaviors and to trigger meaningful responses or interventions. We are also working towards establishing a new standard of suicide prevention care by analyzing measures of Veteran-reported symptoms to tailor mental health treatments to individual needs.

On April 8, 2016, VA leadership strategized to elevate and enhance the Suicide Prevention Program, in order to ensure that VA is able to fulfill ongoing and new suicide prevention initiatives. Plans are underway to elevate VA's Suicide Prevention Program with additional resources and a new reporting structure in order to strengthen current programs and initiatives.

In addition, to continue our commitment to preventing deaths, intentional or inadvertent, from opioid overdoses, every VA facility provides naloxone, which prevents death by overdose. More than 20,000 kits have been provided to Veterans across VA. Veterans and families have been instructed in their use. Educating VA physicians about the importance of ensuring patients only have access to medications they need is essential to decreasing overprescribing.

**Veterans Crisis Line**

VA is committed to ensuring the safety of Veterans, but especially when they are in crisis. We have universal access for 24/7 emergency care through our Emergency Departments and VA's Veterans Crisis Line (1–800–273–TALK (8255), press 1, and www.veteranscrisisline.net). We know that when we diagnose and treat people, they get better. August 2015 marked 8 years since the establishment of VA's Veterans Crisis Line (VCL), which has expanded to include a Chat Service and texting option for contacting the Crisis Line. The program continues to save lives and link Veterans with effective ongoing mental health services on a daily basis.

The Military Crisis Line has also been added, branded to reach active duty service members. Since 2007, the VCL has answered over two million calls, nearly 490,000 of those during the last fiscal year. VCL has made over 267,000 chat connections and communicated with over 48,000 texts. VCL initiated the dispatch of emergency services to callers in imminent suicidal crisis over 11,000 times last year and over

57,000 times total. Finally, the VCL provided over 340,000 referrals to a VA Suicide Prevention Coordinator (SPC) ensuring Veterans are connected to local care.

To address this increased demand, many steps are currently underway. First among these is an increase in responders to 310 Full Time Employee Equivalent . Since January 1, 2016, VCL has brought on 29 administrative personnel to augment areas such as analytics, knowledge management, quality assurance, and training. In addition, 38 new responders have been brought on board during this same period of time, with another 23 in active and ongoing recruitment. New responders are also receiving newly developed training that will allow them to provide the best experience and services to Veterans. This training includes approximately 20 modules, both in person and online, on a wide variety of topics in crisis intervention, substance use disorders, Screening, Brief Intervention, and Referral to Treatment (SBIRT), motivational interviewing, and suicide prevention. In addition, training is now being implemented onsite by dedicated training staff who are all former VCL responders.

The Veterans Crisis Line continues to uphold their extraordinary commitment to Veterans in crisis, demonstrating a 97% satisfaction rating, reported by Veterans who call the VCL and complete an end-of-call survey. In an effort to further improve the quality of the Veteran experience at VCL, Quality assurance processes have been initiated. These began April 3 with the selection of six dedicated silent monitors. This along with recruitment of a Quality Management Officer expected to be on board by May 15, 2016 will bring VCL in line with Quality Management processes that are considered best in industry practices

## Expanding Mental Health Services

While focusing on suicide prevention, we know that preventing suicide for the population we serve does not begin with an intervention as someone is about to take an action that could end his or her life. We are aware of how we work to prevent fatal heart attacks. We must similarly focus on prevention, which includes addressing many factors that contribute to someone feeling suicidal. We are aware that access to mental health care is one significant part of preventing suicide. VA is determined to address systemic problems with access to care in general and to mental health care, including substance use disorders in particular. VA has recommitted to a culture that puts the Veteran first. To serve the growing number of Veterans seeking mental health care, VA has deployed significant resources and increased staff in mental health services. Between 2005 and 2015, the number of Veterans who received mental health care from VA grew by eighty percent. This rate of increase is more than three times that seen in the overall number of VA users over the same time period. This reflects VA's concerted efforts to engage Veterans who are new to our system and stimulate better access to mental health services for Veterans within our system. In addition, this reflects VA's efforts to eliminate barriers to receiving mental health care, including the stigma associated with receiving mental health care and treatment for substance use disorders.

Easing the way Veterans receive care from mental health providers also has allowed more Veterans to receive care. VA Telemental Health innovations provided more than 380,000 encounters to over 122,000 Veterans in 2015. Telemental Health reaches Veterans where and when they are best served. VA is a leader across the US and internationally in these efforts. VA's MaketheConnection.net, Suicide Prevention campaigns, and the Posttraumatic Stress Disorder (PTSD) mobile app (which has been downloaded over 208,000 times) contribute to increasing Mental Health access and utilization. VA has also created a suite of award-winning tools that can be utilized as self-help resources or as an adjunct to active mental health services and substance use disorders.

Additionally, in 2007, VA began national implementation of integrated mental health services in primary care clinics. Primary Care-Mental Health Integration (PC–MHI) services include both co-located collaborative functions and evidence-based care management, a telephone based modality of care. By co-locating mental health providers within primary care clinics, Veterans are able to be introduced same day by their primary care team to a mental health provider present in the clinic, thereby reducing wait times and no show rates for mental health services. Additionally, integration of mental health providers within primary care has been shown to improve the identification of mental health disorders and substance use disorders and increase the rates of treatment. Several studies of the program have also shown that treatment within PC–MHI increases the odds of attending future mental health appointments and engaging in specialty mental health treatment. Finally, the integration of primary care and mental health has shown consistent improvement of quality of care and outcomes, including patient satisfaction. The PC–MHI program continues to expand and through December 2015, has provided over

5.5 million PC–MHI clinic encounters, serving over 1.3 million individuals since October 1, 2007.

These efforts align with VA's interagency activities including the Cross Agency Priority (CAP) Goals and expanding VA mental health policy and practice. We anticipate that demand for VA mental health care, including treatment for substance use disorders, will continue to grow as active duty personnel separate from service. Importantly, in an effort to help Veterans who have not enrolled in VA for care, these applications are important lifelines to understanding their symptoms and helping them to overcome other barriers to care.

### VA Mental Health Services and Suicide Prevention for Women Veterans

VA conducts annual, comprehensive assessments of suicide deaths that occur among Veterans using VA health services. These assessments evaluate gender differences in suicide rates. While the suicide rate among women Veterans are lower than the rate in male Veterans, suicide rate among women Veterans have increased in recent years.

Providing high-quality care specific to women Veterans is a priority and VA offers a full continuum of mental health services to women Veterans. Evidence-based therapies for PTSD, including prolonged exposure and cognitive processing therapy, have been shown to decrease suicidal ideation. These treatments are available at every VA medical center. Women Veterans have access to comprehensive mental health services at every VA medical center. VA has residential and inpatient programs that provide treatment to women only or, that have separate tracks for women and men. These residential and inpatient programs are considered regional and/or national resources, not just a resource for the local VA facility. VA remains committed to ensuring that appropriate services are available to meet the treatment needs of women (and men) Veterans who have experienced Military Sexual Trauma (MST) and may be at risk for suicide.

### Breakthrough Outcomes for 2016

We are looking to achieve three breakthrough outcomes for 2016. First, we remain focused to increasing access to health care. When Veterans call for a new mental health appointment, they receive a suicide risk assessment and immediate care, if needed. Veterans already engaged in mental health care identifying a need for urgent attention will speak with a provider the same day. Second, we will modernize our Contact Centers, including the Veterans Crisis Line. Veterans will have a single toll free phone number to access the VA Contact Centers, know where to call to get their questions answered, receive prompt service and accurate answers, and be treated with kindness and respect. By the end of this year, every Veteran in crisis will have his or her call promptly answered by an experienced responder at the Veterans Crisis Line. Third, we will staff critical positions. VA is looking to achieve significantly improved critical staffing levels that balance access and clinical productivity. This will increase the rate at which positions are filled.

Timely access to mental health care for our Veterans is of utmost importance to VA. We acknowledge that we have work to do in this area, and we are constantly working to increase access. We are in partnerships with other Federal agencies, community providers, and through the use of tele-mental health, we are increasing access. There are many entry points for mental health care, including 168 VA medical centers, 1,035 Community Based Outpatient Clinics and Outpatient Services sites, 300 Vet Centers providing readjustment counseling, 80 Mobile Vet Centers, a national Veterans Crisis Line, VA staff on college and university campuses, and a variety of other outreach efforts.

### Community Provider Pilot Program

In 2013, 12 VA Medical Centers (VAMCs) developed agreements with 24 Community Mental Health Clinics (CMHCs) across the country to establish Community Mental Health (CMH) pilots. These pilots were created in response to section 3(a) of Executive Order 13625, "Improving Access to Mental Health Services for Veterans, Service Members, and Military Families," which focused on the creation of "Enhanced Partnerships between the Department of Veterans Affairs and Community Providers" designed specifically to decrease wait times and assist in areas where VA has faced challenges in hiring and placing mental health providers. Pilot sites were able to select a model of care to best meet the needs of local Veterans. All sites used one of two broad approaches: Community Care or VA telemental health (TMH), with most sites choosing to provide Non-VA care to Veterans. Non-VA care uses community providers that are paid by VA. TMH care utilizes technology to deliver mental health services via modalities such as video conferencing and allows for real-time (or "synchronous") encounters between health care providers and patients who are not in the same location. During the VA/Community Mental Health Care Pilot partnerships, TMH services enabled Veterans to receive care at designated community clinics that were closer to their homes than the nearest VA medical facilities or clinics.

VA and CMHC staff worked together in determining roles and responsibilities within each pilot partnership. Partnerships using telemental health required space, equipment, a technician, and a protocol for handling emergencies (e.g., a Veteran becoming distressed during a TMH session). For Non-VA care partnerships, there were other responsibilities that needed to be addressed: coordination of care (between VA and CMHCs), billing, and payment. While some pilot site VAMCs developed strong systems for coordinating care, monitoring patients, and billing, other sites, especially smaller ones, experienced challenges in these areas.

Evaluation of the pilots included both gathering data from not only Veterans about their experiences, but also from key staff at each of the participating Veterans Integrated Service Networks (VISN) and VA Central Office (VACO) and a review of key documents associated with the pilots. Results from follow up surveys indicate that Veterans were very satisfied with the services they received via these pilots. When the pilots concluded, each participating VAMC was allowed to determine whether to continue the partnership.

## Additional Efforts to Improve Access

VA has also moved to Patient Centered Community Care, a centralized contracting mechanism, and has implemented the Veterans Choice Program. Regardless of how such care is provided, the growing need for mental health services for Veterans will increase the need for efficient leveraging of Non-VA community providers when access to care is not available within the VA system of care. VA is rising to the challenge through its Community Mental Health Summit program which engaged over 11,000 individuals at 144 sites in FY 14 and continues annually to bring together DoD, VA, State, and Community providers and stakeholders for vital conversations at the local level.

VA and DoD developed a joint Military Cultural Competence Training Program as part of the Integrated Mental Health Strategy which is now housed on the public facing TRAIN website, vha.train.org, and which, to date, has provided free training to over 2,000 providers. Whether mental health care is delivered directly by Non-VA mental health care providers, through TMH care at Non-VA sites, or any other means, it is critical for VA to continue to provide Veterans with access to high quality mental health care in coordination with other VA services.

In addition, VA is addressing access through the following efforts:

- Veteran-centered operating hours: Extended hours help increase capacity when space is limited and improve the match between available staff hours and the needs of Veterans who are employed or have other competing responsibilities during day-time hours.
- Leveraging trainees and fellows: These professionals provide substantial amounts of clinical care under the direct supervision of appropriately licensed and privileged mental health staff. Training programs also provide ready access to well-qualified candidates for recruitment into vacant positions.
- Support staff, adjunct professions, and peer support staff: VA has hired over 900 peer specialists and is developing a pilot program in response to the President's August 2014 Executive Actions to expand the role of peer specialists into primary care settings.

VA's efforts to increase access to mental health care for Veterans face many challenges. These include overcoming stigmas that Veterans may associate with seeking care for mental health, the need to address co-occurring substance use disorders, and fears that associated medical records documenting their care may have an adverse impact on their lives. Additionally, VA struggles to attain and retain a sufficient mental health workforce capacity, establish a competency-based practice, and have adequate systems to support improving care nationwide. In the face of these challenges, we continue to focus our efforts on ensuring Veterans receive timely access to mental health care.

## Hiring Practices

In 2012, VA began a two-part hiring initiative under Executive Order 13625 issued in August 2012. The first part focused on recruiting 1,600 new mental health professionals, 300 new non-clinical support staff (such as scheduling clerks), and filling existing vacancies as of June 2012. The second part was the hiring of 800 peer specialist positions by December 31, 2013. As a result of this initiative, VA hired approximately 5,300 new clinical and non-clinical mental health staff. VA hired 932 peer specialists as well. The Government Accountability Office found that VAMC officials reported local improvements due to the additional hiring, such as more evidence-based therapies offered, mental health care provided at new locations, and a variety of benefits provided by the new peer specialists such as modeling effective coping, engaging Veterans who are resistant to discussing mental health issues, and providing peer-to-peer counseling.

VAMC officials also cited several challenges to hiring mental health care providers such as pay disparity with the private sector, competition among VAMCs, the lengthy hiring process, lack of space and support staff, and an underlying nationwide shortage of mental health professionals. VA has increased its mental health hiring through outreach events at medical schools, through Mental Health professional groups and other means of active recruitment in order to develop the workforce needed to meet the needs of our Veterans who need mental health care. At a national level, VA outpatient mental health staff totals increased from 11,138 full-time equivalents in 2010 to more than 14,000 in FY 2015. Over the same time period, the number of Veterans receiving outpatient mental health care increased from 1,259,300 to more than 1,600,000.

The recent rapid growth in the number of Veterans seeking mental health treatment in VA has posed challenges in the area of staffing. In Figure 1 below, the solid black line shows the growth in numbers of Veterans using mental health services, from 897,600 in 2005 to more than 1,600,000 in 2015. The number of patients is expressed in terms of hundreds to show staff and patient numbers on the same graph. For example, 10,000 on the vertical axis represents 1,000,000 patients and 10,000 full time equivalents employees (FTEs).

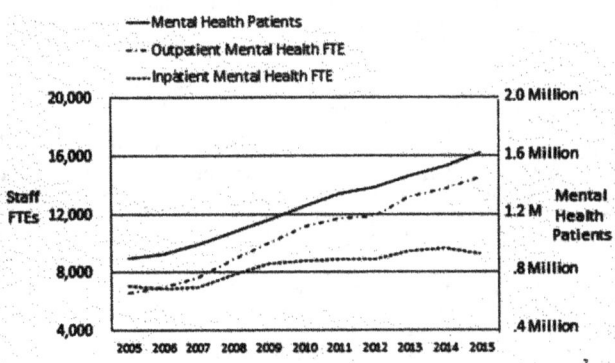

Figure 1. Growth in annual numbers of patients using mental health services and in outpatient and inpatient FTE levels, 2005 to 2014.

This graph also shows the growth in numbers of mental health clinical staff, measured in terms of the FTE providing outpatient and inpatient treatment. Consistent with a shift to outpatient care, the inpatient mental health FTEs began to level off after 2009. Outpatient mental health FTEs began to lag behind the growth in patient numbers in 2012, but as part of the President's 2012 Executive Order 13625, VA hired more than 1,600 new clinical providers by the June 30, 2013, target date.

In the absence of any national benchmark related to mental health staffing, VA continues to refine our model that is intended to inform local facility decision-making about the number of staff necessary to meet local demand for mental health services.

**Clay Hunt Implementation Accomplishments**

The Clay Hunt Suicide Prevention for American Veterans Act (Public Law 114–2) gives VA additional authority to advance suicide prevention efforts for Veterans within the Department and in partnership with the community. As of March, 2016, VA has taken steps to implement each of its requirements, including the Call to Action collaboration previously discussed. To conduct an independent evaluation of

Mental Health and suicide prevention programs, VA has contracted with an independent third party, Enterprise Resource Performance, Inc. (ERPI). VA mental health program evaluation centers are collecting self-report outcome data from Veterans newly receiving mental health care. Funding has been provided to cover the programs included in the Clay Hunt evaluations. The Program Evaluation Centers will support ERPI's request for data to conduct the independent evaluation. The full report by ERPI is due to Congress in 2018, and the first VA interim report that provides descriptive data on specific mental health programs is due in September of 2016. The Office of Mental Health Operation (OMHO) is working with the independent 3rd party evaluator to ensure coordination for these reports.

We are working towards the publication of a website that provides easily-accessible information about mental health services for Veterans. The current VA Facility Locator tool includes information regarding PTSD, Substance Use Disorder, and Vet Center programs and contact and resource information. This tool is currently accessible on several sites, including the VA homepage, VA Mental Health page, and the Make the Connection website. The vets.gov team has developed a prototype for a website to provide a facility locator that includes both services and facilities for Veterans. VA product team and mental health subject matter experts are reviewing the prototype with a planned launch of these enhancements on vets.gov in fall 2016 (Note: this capability is dependent on the existence and availability of required VA data. The VA team is currently working to determine if the necessary data will be available for this enhancement).

To address critical VA health care workforce needs in the area of mental health, VA is establishing a pilot program for the repayment of educational loans (PREL) for certain psychiatrists seeking employment in VA. The program secures a service commitment to a VA health care facility from program participants who are either licensed or eligible for licensure to practice who are enrolled in their final year of a post-graduate physician residency program leading to either a specialty qualification in psychiatric medicine or a subspecialty qualification of psychiatry. In return, VA will pay up to $30,000 a year in qualifying student loan debt for each year of obligated service.

VA has also developed a pilot program using community outreach and peer support to engage Veterans in care. Five Veterans Integrated Service Networks (VISNs), 6, 7, 16, 17, and 22, began implementing the pilot program, with support from the VISN 3 VA Mental Illness Research, Education Clinical Center to conduct the program evaluation component of this initiative.

VA has also implemented an expanded period of eligibility for recent combat Veterans. This resulted in the new enrollment of about 995 Veterans who discharged between January 1, 2009, and January 1, 2011, and who did not enroll in the VA health care during their initial 5 year period of eligibility.

**Legislative Priorities**

VA is grateful for your continuing support of Veterans and appreciates your efforts to pass legislation enabling VA to provide Veterans with the high-quality care they have earned and deserve. As the Department focuses on ways to help provide access to health care across the country, we have identified a number of necessary legislative items that require action by Congress in order to best serve Veterans.

Flexible budget authority would allow VA to avoid artificial restrictions that impede our delivery of care and benefits to Veterans. Currently, there are over 70 line items in VA's budget that dedicate funds to a specific purpose without adequate flexibility to provide the best service to Veterans. These include limitations within the same general areas, such as health care funds that cannot be spent on health care needs and funding that can be used for only one type of Care in the Community program, but not others. These restrictions limit the ability of VA to deliver Veterans with care and benefits based on demand, rather than specific funding lines.

VA also requests your support for legislation that would allow VA to enter into agreements with providers on an individual basis in the community outside of Federal Acquisition Regulations, and includes explicit protections for procurement integrity, provider qualifications, price reasonableness and employment protections. Such legislation will ensure that VA is able to provide local care to Veterans in a timely and responsible manner. VA would support language that addresses concerns related to employment nondiscrimination and equal employment protections. We would have strong concerns with any legislative language, such as that currently being considered by this committee that rolls back employment protections. VA further requests your support for our efforts to recruit and retain the very best clinical professionals. These include, for example, flexibility for the Federal work period requirement, which is not consistent with private sector medicine, and special pay authority to help VA recruit and retain the best talent possible to lead our hospitals and health care networks.

**Conclusion**

Mr. Chairman, VA is saddened by the crisis of suicide among Veterans, but committed to the work we have done in implementing and expanding upon the expectations of this Committee. We remain focused on providing the highest quality care our Veterans have earned and deserve and which our Nation trusts us to provide. Our work to effectively treat Veterans who desire or need mental health care continues to be a top priority. We emphasize that we in VA remain committed to preventing Veteran suicide, aware that prevention requires our system-wide support and intervention in preventing precursors of suicide [1]. We appreciate the support of Congress and look forward to responding to any questions you may have.

○

---

[1] https://www.drugabuse.gov/sites/default/files/drugfacts—subabusemilitary.pdf